THE NURSE
LEADER
COACH

Become the Boss No
One Wants to Leave

ROSE O. SHERMAN

The Nurse Leader Coach
Become the Boss No One Wants to Leave

Inquiries about the book should be directed to: roseosherman@outlook.com
Author Website: www.emergingrnleader.com

ISBN 978-1-7329127-0-0

Library of Congress Control Number: 2018914304

Published by:
Rose O. Sherman

Printed in the United States of America

ACKNOWLEDGMENTS

This book has grown out of my work with nurse leaders over the past three decades. I dedicate this work to the many leaders who I have had the privilege to teach and influence. I have learned as much from you as you have from me. My colleagues at both the American Organization of Nurse Executives and the American Nurses Association have given me opportunities to share my leadership work on a national level and I am grateful.

Nurse leaders stand on the shoulders of those who took the time to mentor and guide them. I was fortunate to have many great nurse mentors including the late Marie Basti, Dr. Anne Boykin and Dr. Roxane Spitzer. I would not be where I am today without these three great ladies.

To my family and new grandson John, you have always been terrific in your support of my career and continually inspire me to do better work.

INTRODUCTION

What nurses expect from their leaders is changing. Gone are the days of command and control leadership when staff were expected to be grateful because they had a job. Today's nurses want their leaders to be coaches who will help them to learn and grow as professionals. The nurse leader has become the linchpin in staff recruitment and retention. When nurses don't receive the coaching and feedback that they desire, they will leave as evidenced by high nursing turnover in many healthcare organizations.

Coaching is a different approach to developing the potential of your staff. When you coach, you provide staff with the opportunity to grow and gain expertise through more consistent feedback, counseling and mentoring. The relationship moves from being leader dominated to a partnership with staff. You don't wait until the annual review to discuss areas in need of improvement. The effective manager-coach takes the time to understand the motivations of individual staff, enables optimal performance, encourages professional success and removes barriers to high-level performance. If you perfect your skills as a coach, you can help staff to grow and put them on a path to success and greater ownership of their professional practice. It also makes performance management much easier because your staff will expect regular feedback.

Moving from being a manager to a nurse leader coach requires a different leadership mindset and skillset to add to your leadership toolbox. The key characteristics of a coaching leadership approach include partnership and collaboration versus command and control. A coaching leadership approach involves less time talking and more time listening. Coaching for performance is an ongoing process that becomes easier over time if you commit to doing it. It will make you a better leader. Included in this book are new ideas, action steps and resources to help you do this.

Research indicates that staff highly value managers who adopt a coaching style of managing performance. Yet for many leaders, this will change how they look at their leadership. Any new change in behavior can be challenging until it becomes routine. Give yourself a competitive edge by learning the secrets of how to become a great leader through coaching. Let this book be your roadmap on this journey. If you commit to becoming a nurse leader coach, you will become the boss that no one wants to leave.

Contents

PART 1

BUILDING A COACHING FOUNDATION

"A good coach can change a game.
A great coach can change a life."

JOHN WOODEN

CHAPTER 1

DEVELOP A COACHING MINDSET

I f you are like most nurse leaders, you were selected for a leadership role because you demonstrate great problem-solving skills in your nursing practice. When you became a leader, your natural inclination was to view yourself as a problem fixer because this is how you add value. For many years, this is how traditional nursing leaders have approached their responsibilities and how they have managed their staff. The problem today is that strategies used by traditional managers are no longer working with the changing nursing workforce. Only 23% of new graduates look forward to going to work each day and close to 62% plan to leave their employers within two years. [1] Turnover is on the rise in all healthcare environments, and nurses are not easily replaced in the current growing nursing shortage. As staff needs and workplace expectations change (Figure 1-1), leaders must change as well. [2]

FIGURE 1-1

The Past ⟶	The Future
Focus on what I earn	Focus on purpose in work
My work satisfaction	My development
My boss	My coach
My annual review	Ongoing coaching
My weaknesses	My strengths
My job	My life

Nurse leaders play a vital role in both staff recruitment and retention. Gallup research indicates that 70% of the variance in employee engagement and satisfaction with their work is directly impacted by the actions of managers.[2] Your success in being the type of leader that nurses won't want to leave hinges on your willingness to change your approach to leadership and to develop new skills. Being a manager is no longer enough. Younger nurses want to get ahead in their careers and expect to be coached on how to do this. Coaching is now an essential part of a leadership toolbox. Becoming a leader coach requires a shift in mindset from a traditional manager role, who is performance focused, to a coach who also looks for opportunities to foster professional growth (Figure 1-2). It means refraining from always jumping in to solve the problems of others, and instead helping them to discover their own solutions.[3]

A coaching mindset means moving from a leadership style focused on fixing staff weaknesses to a strengths-based approach focused on helping staff accelerate their professional growth through real-time feedback and communication. There are many situations in the workplace where a coaching approach can be used to help staff reach higher levels of performance by growing their talents and skills. These include situations such as:

FIGURE 1-2

The Traditional Manager	The Leader Coach
Focuses on Performance Only Feedback Only When Needed Corrects Weaknesses Asks – what can I do for you?	Focuses on Professional Growth Provides Frequent Feedback Builds on Strengths Asks – what can we do together?

- Career development
- Performance management
- Skills and competency feedback
- Promoting more effective teamwork
- Relationship management
- Staff well being
- Critical thinking and problem solving
- Motivating and inspiring
- Delegating new areas of responsibility
- Leadership development

Coaching is a collaborative relationship undertaken between the coach and the nurse. It uses conversations to help the nurse plan and achieve their goals and enables higher levels of performance. Moving from being the problem solver in chief who tells others what to do to a coach takes practice. Listening, reflecting on what you hear and sense, and then asking powerful questions can change how a nurse sees themselves and the world around them.

Changing Your Leadership Approach

Bob's story is a good illustration of what can happen when a leader understands and commits to a change in their approach. Bob is a seasoned manager in a large critical care unit. He has 75 nurses who directly report to him. Bob takes great pride in how he manages his unit. He used to say his unit was such a well-oiled machine that it could run on autopilot. However, things changed about three years ago. Bob lost five of his experienced Baby Boomer nurses to retirement. He began to have challenges hiring experienced critical-care nurses. Within a few short years, his unit became a revolving door as his younger nurses came, gained experience and then left. The skills and abilities that led to his selection as the manager of the unit were not serving him as well with younger nurses who sought something different from their manager. Bob was wise enough to realize it.

Bob took the time to meet with each one of his direct reports to talk about their professional needs. This is something that he had never done in his decade as a leader. His previous philosophy was built on his own need for very little feedback where "no news is good news." When he did meet with staff in the past, he did most of the talking and provided direction on what needed to be done. He was determined to change this pattern of communication by listening carefully and asking open-ended questions that required more than a yes or no answer such as:

1. What is working well in our unit?
2. What do you need from me as your leader?
3. What are your unique strengths as a nurse?
4. What changes would you recommend to improve care and the unit environment?
5. What do you want from your career?
6. How can I help you to reach your goals?

Bob learned a great deal from these conversations. In meeting one on one with each of his nurses, he discovered that many said they wanted to "get ahead in their careers." This restless need to "get ahead" was a mystery to Bob. He had spent the first five years of his career working hard to gain clinical skills and had thought little about career advancement outside the unit. When asked about what they needed from him, a common theme from his younger staff was that they wanted more frequent feedback. He soon realized that his team was asking him for coaching.

Coaching was something Bob was familiar with because he was the coach of his son's basketball team. He had never considered applying these concepts to his leadership. Before he had begun coaching his son's team, he had studied some legendary coaches including John Wooden. John Wooden had won ten NCAA national basketball championships in a 12-year period as head coach at UCLA. No other team had won more than two in a row. He was named national coach of the year six times.

What Bob learned from studying Wooden is that he spent more time talking one on one with his players than he ever did in strategizing about the game. He was renowned for his short, simple inspirational messages to his players, including his "Pyramid of Success."[4] These messages were often directed at how to be a success in life as well as in basketball. He defined success as the peace of mind which is a direct result of self-satisfaction in knowing you made an effort to become the best you are capable of becoming. His coaching transformed the lives of his players. Bob recognized he had the potential do to the same for his staff by seeing himself as a leader coach.

THE COACHING PROCESS

To become an effective leader coach, leaders need to draw from best practices in coaching. One of the most widely used coaching models is the GROW Model depicted in Figure 1-3.[5]

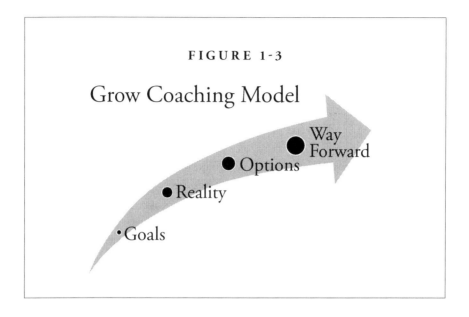

FIGURE 1-3

Grow Coaching Model

Coaching should be thought of as a journey and the following are the steps along the way:

1. **PRE-COACHING ASSESSMENT**

   The focus during this phase is on relationship building and an assessment of needs and opportunities for growth. This is achieved by meeting one to one with staff as Bob did and asking thoughtful open-ended questions. Some staff may have specific goals that they want to achieve, but many may not as Bob found other than wanting to "get ahead." He could ask a question such as *What matters most to you in your career?* to help gain clarity. Other good questions to ask during this phase could include *What would a successful nursing career look like for you?* or *What new skills would you like to learn?*

2. **GROW – ESTABLISH GOALS**

   The second phase in the coaching process is where specific goals and a plan are mutually developed. For Bob, this is where he and his staff discussed some growing in place strategies that his nurses could use at this point in their careers such as becoming certified, joining a unit committee or becoming involved in a professional association. Ask the staff member about their next steps. An effective plan needs to be in writing and formalized with dates/times/activities.

3. **REALITY – EXAMINE WHERE THE STAFF MEMBER CURRENTLY IS IN RELATION TO THE GOALS.**

    Too often, people try to solve a problem or reach a goal without fully considering their starting point. They may be missing some information that they need in order to reach their goal effectively. This is why defining the current reality becomes essential. Questions such as how much personal time a staff member is willing to put in to move their careers forward is important because goals will not happen without some sacrifices.

4. **OPTIONS – EXPLORE THE POSSIBILITIES TO ENSURE THAT THE GOALS ARE REACHED.**

    Bob could offer his assistance, but there must be a mutual commitment to act. What are the obstacles that stand in the way? What is working on the road to achieving these goals? What are some strategies that could be considered to achieve the goals? Are there others who could help to provide insight and guidance? What might the staff member need to stop doing to be more successful?

5. **WAY FORWARD – IDENTIFY THE MOST EFFECTIVE WAYS TO ACHIEVE THE GOALS.**

    This is a phase where progress begins and is tracked and evaluated, and where coaching feedback is provided. During this phase, revisions can be made to the plan and both the leader coach and staff member can provide input on the success of the career coaching. The feedback loop is an essential part of the coaching process. Coaching is not one and done — it is ongoing.

Avoiding Common Coaching Mistakes

Throughout this book, best practices to use in your coaching will be presented. There are also some common coaching mistakes that we will discuss.[6] They include the following:

- *Assuming everyone wants to be coached* – you will learn as a nurse leader coach that not everyone will want to be coached. Two key questions to consider is whether your staff member wants to get better, and are they willing to assume the discomfort of doing things differently. If the answer to these questions is no then your attempts to coach them are unlikely to be successful.
- *Skipping the need to build trust* – the foundation of the coaching relationship is trust, but this does not happen overnight. Trust must be earned in order to build a strong coaching relationship.
- *Trying too hard to be a great coach* – the focus of the coaching conversation should be on listening to staff members that you are coaching and their goals for themselves.
- *Not saying what needs to be said* – some coaching conversations are challenging because you may surface behaviors that the staff member needs to change. These are crucial conversations that need to happen for you to effectively coach. The nurse leader coach must have the courage to initiate these difficult discussions.
- *Neglecting to ask the staff member how you can be most helpful* – when coaching, you want the staff member to own both the agenda and outcomes.
- *Assuming the staff member needs to be "fixed"* – there may be situations where you are coaching to improve performance but to be effective, you must be supportive and believe that the staff member can be successful.
- *Talking too much* – your goal should be to spend the majority of your time in a coaching conversation (75%) attentively listening

versus talking. Become comfortable with silence. Often the most significant breakthroughs happen when you stop talking.

- *Giving too much advice* – the goal in coaching is to help staff reach their own conclusions.
- *Believing that you know what is best for the individual* – you should not own the outcomes of the coaching session. To create ownership of goals, you will need to challenge, affirm and advocate but ultimately the choice to move forward belongs to the staff member being coached.
- *Failing to get a commitment to advance the goals discussed* – every coaching session should end with the staff member committing to goals and a series of action steps. To achieve this, coaches need to build momentum, be encouraging and require goal commitment. [2]
- *Not individualizing your coaching* – coaching is a two-way commitment. While adopting a leader coach style will be embraced by most of your staff, some may resist and want a more traditional management approach.

Coaching Example

Sarah was a new graduate working on Bob's unit. She had just completed her one-year RN residency program. During their one to one session, Sarah told Bob that she felt she had mastered the responsibilities of being a critical care nurse and was ready for the next step in her career. Bob did not agree with Sarah's assessment of her competency level. He felt she had made progress in her clinical knowledge but still had a great deal to learn. In the past, Bob would have jumped in and corrected Sarah's perceptions of her progress urging her to focus on building her clinical skills. With his commitment to being a leader coach, he took a different strategy. They mutually developed a plan that included both clinical skills development and opportunities for Sarah to begin to grow her leadership. He committed to helping her achieve her career goals and scheduled quarterly feedback sessions.

Not every nurse has the same needs for career coaching as Sarah. Some may resist coaching or don't want to move out of their comfort zones. The leader coach must adapt to the needs of individual staff. There are situations where coaching is not the right approach, and telling is more effective such as emergencies. The value of a coaching mindset is that it creates a culture of interdependency versus the dependency that is often seen in traditional management structures. It stems from a leadership value system that believes in the potential, resourcefulness, and capability of both yourself and others.

We have strong evidence today that your leadership approach has a significant impact on staff performance. Coaching is an approach that leads to higher levels of both individual and team performance through the fostering of independence and interdependence. The principles of coaching that we discuss in this book can be effectively applied to most aspects of nursing leadership to bring staff to a higher level of performance and improve staff retention.

Remember

- ✓ A coaching mindset means moving from a leadership style focused on fixing staff weaknesses to a strengths-based approach focused on building the strengths of staff.
- ✓ Moving from being the problem solver in chief who tells others what to do to a coach takes practice.
- ✓ The GROW Model is an evidence-based coaching framework that can be quickly learned.
- ✓ Nurse leader coaches bring staff to higher levels of performance and have lower turnover rates.

CHAPTER 2

MANAGE YOURSELF

To be an effective leader coach, you need to have strong self-management skills. Coaching requires that we suspend judgment and remain openly curious in working with others. In coaching staff, we are working to help them build their own personal mastery. Great coaches need to model behaviors that they seek in others by understanding their values, beliefs, and attitudes. In their book *The Leadership Challenge,* Kouzes and Posner outline over 30 years of research with thousands of employees to study the expectations that followers have of their leaders.[7] They asked for a ranking of 20 different characteristics. Over time, the results are remarkably stable globally. The top four characteristics that followers value most in leaders are:

1. **Honesty** – the leader is principled, ethical and truthful.
2. **Competence** – the leader has a track record and ability to get things done to meet the expectations of the position.

3. **Inspiring** – the leader is excited, energetic and confident about the future. They give their followers hope.
4. **Forward-Looking** – the ability to look ahead and have a sense of direction — a point of view about the future.

When present, these four qualities lead to a concept called *"source credibility."* In their research, Kouzes and Posner found that source credibility matters in leadership. When nursing staff finds their leader to be highly credible, they are more likely to:

- Feel pride that they work on the unit.
- Feel a stronger sense of team spirit.
- See their own personal values as consistent with the organization.
- Feel engaged with the work.
- Have a sense of ownership in the organization.

Leadership credibility is built over time. It also involves a focus on self-mastery. Focusing on self-mastery is often not a high priority when nurses begin in leadership roles. Instead, the majority of time is spent learning core business skills such as budgeting, staffing, and quality management. These skills are critical to effective leadership. However, we know from leadership research that when leaders fail, it is rarely because of a lack of knowledge about business skills. Most leadership performance can be attributed to emotional intelligence (EI) not intelligence quotient (IQ). Self-management is one of the four cornerstones of EI. The other three are self-awareness, social awareness, and relationship management. Leadership coaching is described as an inside-out process. You need to know and understand yourself before you can manage and coach others.

In 1999, Peter F. Drucker (the father of modern management theory) wrote a now classic article for the Harvard Business Review titled *Managing Oneself.*[8] He observed that there are few naturally great achievers in life and that most of us will need to learn to manage ourselves to be successful. Here are four strategies to better manage yourself adapted from Drucker's thinking on this subject:

1. **KNOW YOUR STRENGTHS AND YOUR OWN PERSONALITY**
   Drucker observed that most people are not that good at identifying their own strengths and weaknesses. He was an early proponent of the concept of strengths-based leadership. There are many ways of discovering our strengths that we will discuss in a later chapter. It is also important to recognize that each individual, yourself included, has different personality traits. In this chapter, we will discuss a commonly referenced psychological framework that is easily remembered as OCEAN.

2. **IDENTIFY HOW YOU GET THINGS DONE**
   Nurse leaders often struggle in managing their work. Most don't take the time to analyze how they get their job done. Leaders should be aware of their learning style. Do you absorb information better by reading or listening? Understanding your personal work habits is critical. As an example, do you work better alone or with others? Knowing whether your peak performance is in the morning or the later in the afternoon can also help you more effectively structure your work.

3. **UNDERSTAND YOUR VALUES**
   Your personal values should be the ultimate litmus test on whether a job is the right one for you or not. Does the organization's culture, mission, and strategic direction align with what you believe is essential in your work? They don't need to be the same but they do need to be close enough to co-exist. When your values are in conflict, it can be impossible to do your best work and support the goals of your organization.

4. **Figure out where you belong**

Figuring out where you belong in the world can be a challenge. Some roles are a great fit with our strengths and talents, and others are not. Many nurses are not comfortable in leadership roles and would prefer to work more closely with patients. Recognizing this to be true about yourself requires courage and insight.

Understanding the Personality Puzzle

Great coaches understand that each individual (themselves included) has unique personality traits that need to be honored in the relationship. One easy-to-remember model, often termed OCEAN in the field of psychology, was developed by Dr. Lewis Goldberg. It has five factors that are measured on a sliding scale from high to low:[9] They include the following:

Openness – This personality trait reflects how you approach new ideas and change. It also describes your curiosity and creativity. If you are very open, you enjoy change and pursuing new ideas. If you are less open, you value routines and traditions.

Conscientiousness – This trait describes your approach to getting things done. It measures your self-discipline, organizational skills, and reliability. If you are very conscientious, you probably keep to-do lists and enjoy detailed work. If you are less conscientious, you probably prefer working on big-picture projects and strategy. You may find schedules stifling and may not worry as much about delivering on goals you have set.

Extroversion – This personality trait involves how you approach people. Do social situations energize you or do they exhaust you?

If you are extroverted, you get energy from being with others and seek out social time. If you are introverted, you probably value your alone time and may find social events draining.

Agreeableness – This trait describes how you approach cooperation and working with others. It also speaks to your empathy and willingness to forgive others. If you are agreeable, you are usually more empathetic and quickly forgive the mistakes of others. If you are less agreeable, you are more analytical, practical and keep emotion out of decisions.

Neuroticism – This personality trait describes how you approach worry and how reactive you are to changes in your environment. If you are neurotic, you may worry about every situation. If you are less neurotic, you worry less and are more stabilized in your moods.

Personality plays a significant role in how we make decisions, handle responsibilities and form goals. As a coach, you need to decode your personality before you work with others because it has a strong influence on your coaching. The five-factor OCEAN model is a roadmap for assessing your personality and those of others.

WHY **EI** MATTERS MORE THAN **IQ** IN LEADERSHIP COACHING

In the past when leadership candidates were selected, the focus was on the candidate's competence and intelligence. Today, we know that it is EI and not IQ that separates outstanding leaders from the rest. It is our EI that affects how we coach others, negotiate complex social situations and make decisions. As a nurse leader coach, we guide others to higher levels of self-awareness. To do this, it is essential that we ourselves are self-aware, have good self-management skills and foster and maintain good relationships with others.

Emotional intelligence was popularized in 1995 by Daniel Goleman with the publication of his best-selling book on the topic. [10] Emotional intelligence is defined as self-mastery or the ability to understand and control what we feel (our emotions) and the way we act (our response to these emotions). It is about self-awareness, self-management, social-awareness and relationship management. These four components of EI can be defined as follows:

- **Self-awareness** – You recognize your own emotions and how they affect your thoughts and behavior. You know your strengths and weaknesses and have self-confidence.
- **Self-management** – You can control impulsive feelings and behaviors. You can manage your emotions in healthy ways, take initiative, follow through on commitments, and adapt to changing circumstances.
- **Social awareness** – You can understand the emotions, needs, and concerns of other people, pick up on emotional cues, feel comfortable socially, and recognize the power dynamics in a group or organization.
- **Relationship management** – You know how to develop and maintain good relationships. You communicate clearly, inspire and influence others, work well in a team, and manage conflict.

Marshall Goldsmith, an executive leadership coach, has identified specific behaviors that leaders may exhibit when they have challenges with these four areas of emotional intelligence. He describes them as derailers. [11] They include the following:

1. **Adding too much value**

   Nurse leaders sometimes feel compelled to comment on every situation, add their opinions to every conversation or they wordsmith every document they are given to review. Adding too much value is a common problem in leadership and makes one less effective as a coach. It is a behavior that our co-workers and team will find annoying when done to excess. I once had a colleague who was aware that she tended to dominate group discussions with her opinions. When this was brought to her attention, she developed a plan to stop this behavior by wearing a rubber band at meetings. She used the rubber band as a trigger to stop and ask whether the comment she was about to make would add value to the conversation. Learning when to say nothing and let others talk is a skill that many leaders need to develop. Before you make a remark that you may later regret, ask yourself whether what you are about to say is true, is necessary and is strategic.

2. **Passing judgment**

   Many good ideas are never implemented because nurse leaders are too quick to pass judgment on the idea or the person. Staff will stop offering suggestions if they feel that their leader shuts down the discussion. This can happen when nurse leaders pass judgment on the values, beliefs, and attitudes of their diverse workforce without trying to understand the viewpoints of others.

3. **Passing the buck**

   Some nurse leaders present changes in policies or procedures as decisions that are entirely outside of their control imposed by out of touch administrators. There may be a good rationale for changes, but this is not discussed with staff. Interestingly leaders who do this are often viewed as being powerless in the eyes of their team.

4. Starting with "no", "but", or "however"

Some leaders shut down discussions when they use words such as no, but or however when responding to a different viewpoint. The message conveyed is not that there is simply a difference in opinion but rather the other person is wrong. Leaders should monitor their conversations to see how often they use the words no, but or however.

5. Speaking when angry

Emotional volatility is not a good management tool. Nurse leaders need to control their anger even in difficult conversations. Leadership reputations can be severely damaged when leaders have an angry emotional response to a situation. It is far better to say nothing or walk away from the other person than to say something you will later regret.

6. Withholding information

Some nurse leaders falsely believe that information is power. This can work in the short run to maintain an advantage over someone else but it rarely works in the long run. Withholding information breeds distrust. In today's environment, younger generations of nurses look for transparency and want information shared with them. Sharing information will make you a more powerful leader.

7. Failing to give proper recognition

Nursing staff wants to be valued for their contributions to the work of the team. When leaders fail to say thank you or when they take the recognition for themselves, staff feel devalued. Successful people become great leaders when they shift the focus from themselves to others.

8. Playing favorites

It is natural that nurse leaders may feel closer to some staff than others. What is important as a leader is to be fair and to discourage behaviors that appear to others as "fawning over you" to engender favoritism. Sometimes nurse leaders play favorites with staff that are not their top performers. This tilts the field against honest, principled employees who won't play along.

9. Multitasking instead of listening

Nurse leaders have extremely challenging and busy roles. The most passive-aggressive form of disrespect for a staff member is to continue multitasking (reading email, answering phone calls) when they try to have an important conversation with you. An interesting thing about listening is that people don't notice when you do it but are certainly aware of when you are not listening.

10. Failing to express gratitude

Thank you is a magical gesture that some nurse leaders don't use enough. There is nothing more disheartening to staff than to work short-staffed and hear nothing from their leader. An attitude of gratitude is important in leadership.

When a nurse leader coach lacks emotional intelligence, it can result in higher staff turnover, reduced engagement, poor relationships with other departments and an unhealthy work environment. Managers who struggle with emotional intelligence and other behaviors described above often derail early in their careers.

This almost happened to Jackie in her first leadership position. As part of a leadership development program, she participated in a 360-degree leadership assessment that involved self, supervisor, and direct reports as well as peer feedback. Jackie was shocked to learn that others did not share her self-perceptions about her leadership. She was viewed as smart but often arrogant in her approach and not receptive to feedback. While deeply hurt initially, Jackie chose to use the input to develop a plan to work on her emotional intelligence. The results from a follow-up 360-degree evaluation one year later indicated that Jackie had made significant progress and that it was visible to others.

Like Jackie, you can grow in your emotional intelligence skills as a leader, and avoid letting our emotions hijack your behavior. Here are some examples of actions you can take to assess your own emotional intelligence and potential problem areas:

1. Seek feedback on your behavior to determine how you are perceived by others.
2. Evaluate all negative feedback and reactions to your behavior to look for evidence of where you may have problems with EI.
3. Self-reflect on how you have managed your emotions in highly charged situations with conflict and ask yourself whether there is room for improvement?
4. Assess how you manage your stress level and whether this interferes with relationships with others.
5. Do cognitive rehearsals when confronted with difficult situations to plan how you will manage if you are losing control of the situation.

In many coaching situations with staff, difficulties with emotional intelligence can sometimes be at the core of challenges. Developing your emotional intelligence takes intentionality. Saying *"This is just who I am"* will not lead to growth. Instead when you do make a mistake, step back and ask yourself what you will do differently in future situations. Remember—your leadership success and ability to coach others are highly dependent on your level of emotional intelligence.

Reflecting on your Leadership

In the leader coach role, you will often be asking staff to reflect on their goals and work. Leaders often leave little time in their daily work to reflect on their own leadership. When confronted with challenges, leaders will stay in motion and keep putting out the fires. Real learning from our experiences requires reflection. Until we reflect on situations looking at our behaviors and actions, we may not develop the new insights needed to lead us to act differently in the future. Instead of constant acceleration, we need to at times just stop and think.

Kendra is an excellent example of how much can be learned from reflecting on a challenging situation. She hastily accepted a new leadership role in her organization because it appeared to be a fast track promotion. Three months into the role, she realized that she was working for a toxic leader. She was extremely upset about her situation. Her mentor urged her to reflect for a few days on what she had learned. After thinking about the whole experience, she identified the following key learnings:

1. She had jumped at an opportunity without doing the due diligence needed to assess if it was a good fit.
2. She had been flattered that this leader would consider her for this role with minimal experience.
3. She had not sought out the guidance of mentors who had been helpful to her in the past.
4. She was naïve in workplace politics and assessing the leadership style of others.

These were significant insights for a young leader on her career journey. It is essential to examine events and ask ourselves how they have shaped the way we see the world, others and ourselves. The act of reflection can help build our resiliency. It offers us the opportunity to go back and think through what we would do differently the next time instead of ruminating about the outcomes of our actions. It is proactive versus reactive thinking and helps us to do more proactive reflective thinking in the future.

Some leaders, especially in the early stages of a new role, find reflective journaling to be helpful. The act of writing down your ideas can help to clarify thinking. The following three-step framework is recommended to evaluate challenging experiences: [12]

1. Describe the experience or event – Tell the story of what happened as objectively as possible, sticking to the facts. Include key details such as who was involved, where it happened and when it happened.

2. Express your reaction to what happened – Document your response to the event or experience as factually and objectively as possible. Answer questions such as how you responded, and what your thoughts and your emotional feelings were.

3. Identify your lessons learned – Assess what you learned from both the event and your reaction to it. Have you identified some development needs that you might have in order to better cope with such incidents in the future? Is there a pattern in the way you react to events? What would you do differently if the situation occurred again?

Increasingly, we now see reflection being added to leadership competency models. Your leadership experiences are only as valuable as what you do with them, and this requires reflection. It is a skill that you will also want to recommend to the staff that you coach.

CLARIFY YOUR CORE VALUES

To have self-awareness in your leadership coaching, it is important to know what you believe in and value as a leader. In their book, *The Leadership Challenge,* Kouzes, and Posner identify clarifying one's values as one of the five exemplary practices of great leaders.[7] By identifying those principles that matter most, you will gain tremendous clarity and focus that will allow you to make consistent decisions and take committed action. You will also be a much more effective coach.

Leaders who have clear leadership philosophies and values are rated 40% higher on their leadership skills than those who don't have clear values. Finding your voice as a leader allows you to more effectively choose a direction, act with determination and make the tough choices that come with leadership roles, and more effectively coach others to understand their own values. Values should constitute your personal "bottom line." They help you decide when to say no and when to say yes. The clearer that you are about your values, the easier it will be to stay on your chosen path and commit to it. Some examples of nurse leader coach's core values could include:

- A commitment to collaboration and teamwork
- A belief in the need to foster innovation
- A willingness to tolerate differences in opinions
- A commitment to the patient experience
- A commitment to coach and develop staff
- A belief in a strengths-based approach to leadership

In a coaching relationship, your ability to remain objective is one of the greatest gifts you can give to your staff. It can become a bridge to greater insight. To achieve objectivity, personal mastery is a crucial beginning step.

REMEMBER

- ✓ To be an effective leader coach, you need to have strong self-management skills.
- ✓ Great coaches understand that each individual has unique personality traits that need to be honored in the relationship.
- ✓ Emotional intelligence matters more than IQ in leadership coaching.
- ✓ Until we reflect on situations looking at our own behaviors and actions, we may not develop the new insights needed to make us more effective leader coaches.

CHAPTER 3

BUILD TRUST

Trust is the foundation of building a coaching relationship with your staff. Without trust, leaders lose their ability to influence and retain nurses. It is not built overnight. In his book *The Seven Habits of Highly Effective People,* the late Stephen Covey talked about *the emotional piggy bank* (Figure 3-1).[13] This is an excellent way for nurse leaders to think about trust in their work settings. If as a leader, I make deposits with you in this emotional bank account through courtesy, kindness, honesty and keeping my commitments then I build a reserve. Your trust in me grows and I can call upon that trust when I need it. When trust is high, communication is easier and more effective. If instead as a leader, I show a lack of concern, disrespect, failure to follow-through on commitments or overreact in situations then my emotional bank account can quickly become overdrawn. You won't trust me. Trust requires frequent deposits. If I do make mistakes as a leader but I have large deposits in the emotional bank account, then you will be more likely to forgive me. Research from Gallup indicates that to have a high level of trust, managers need to make six deposits for every withdrawal. [2]

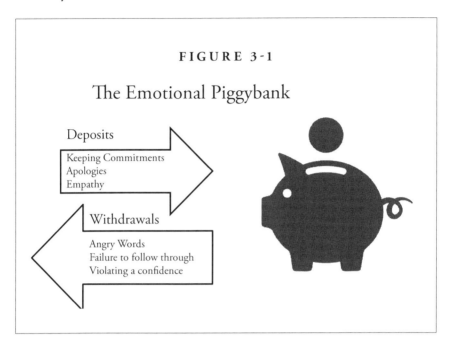

FIGURE 3-1

The Emotional Piggybank

Deposits

Keeping Commitments
Apologies
Empathy

Withdrawals

Angry Words
Failure to follow through
Violating a confidence

Consistency in your leadership actions is key to building trust. Think of it as an equation: **Leadership Trust = Consistency in Leadership Practice divided by Time**. New leaders are often surprised that staff may not trust them but trust does not happen immediately. It is instead like a forest that grows over time but can be burned down with acts of carelessness. The lower the trust, the more time everything takes the more everything costs, and the lower the loyalty of everyone involved. Nurse leader coaches should focus on the creation of trust as an explicit objective. You need to recognize that in healthcare environments, trust impacts the quality of every relationship, every communication, every work project and every effort that the nursing team engages in.

In *The Trust Edge,* Horsager identified eight pillars of trust that are key attributes of successful leaders: [14]

1. Clarity – People trust the clear and mistrust the ambiguous.
2. Compassion – People put faith in those who care beyond themselves.
3. Character – People notice those who do what is right over what is easy.
4. Competency – People have confidence in those who stay fresh, relevant, and capable.
5. Commitment – People believe in those who stand through adversity.
6. Connection – People want to follow, buy from, and be around friends.
7. Contribution – People immediately respond to results.
8. Consistency – People love to see the little things done consistently.

When Trust Is Broken

Mending a broken trust can be challenging. Kara learned this lesson when she took a manager position on a medical-surgical unit that had three previous managers leave in a four-year period. As part of her first 100-day transition plan to her new role, she met with each of her direct reports. She was enthusiastic about her new role and felt confident from her previous leadership experience that she could turn around a unit culture that was characterized by poor morale and disengagement.

What surprised her was the level of suspicion that nurses had about her desire to be a coach and work with them on their development. Kara soon realized that the foundation to begin her coaching with the staff was not there.

Kara's experience is not unusual if you accept a leadership role where previous leaders stayed for only short periods of time. To have real impact in a leadership role, it takes time to build the trust and confidence of staff that you will do what you say you will do. To rebuild trust, Kara should acknowledge the feelings of her team and commit to earning their trust back. Trust is the currency of leadership, and it will be challenging to move forward without rebuilding it. Over time as she makes deposits into the emotional piggybanks of staff, she can earn it back.

CREATING A ZONE OF PSYCHOLOGICAL SAFETY

Another critical element in coaching is the creation of a zone of psychological safety for staff. Dr. Amy Edmondson is an expert on psychological safety in the workplace. She provides the following description: "psychological safety describes the individuals' perceptions about the consequences of interpersonal risk in their work environment." [14] It consists of taken-for-granted beliefs about how others will respond when you put yourself on the line, such as by asking a question, seeking feedback, reporting a mistake, or proposing a new idea. We weigh each potential action against a particular interpersonal climate, as in, *"If I do this here, will I be hurt, embarrassed or criticized?"* An action that might be unthinkable in one workgroup can be readily taken in another, due to different beliefs about probable interpersonal consequences.

A lack of psychological safety in the work environment was the challenge that Maria encountered as a new director in the emergency department. Her predecessor had exercised a command and control approach to leadership. Blame and incivility were characteristics of the culture that had evolved over many years. New graduate turnover was very high because of the lack of support from experienced staff leaving new nurses with feelings of failure during their professional transition.

Maria was a natural leader coach but felt staff resistance to any of her attempts at coaching. The previous manager had managed staff by focusing on their weaknesses. When mistakes were made, it was held against the staff member who made the error. During staff meetings, she had noticed that staff were reluctant to voice their opinions. In her interviews with staff, few suggestions for unit improvement were offered.

Maria understood that to move the staff to a higher level of performance, she needed first to build a zone of psychological safety. She could not re-engage staff unless they felt comfortable discussing challenges and did not fear retribution. On a team where members feel psychological safety, staff has confidence that they will receive respect and consideration from others. On a team with a culture of psychological safety, the leader encourages open discussion of tough issues. He or she not only tolerates disagreement but also nurtures contrasting points of view. To rebuild a zone of psychological safety, Maria presented for discussion new unit core values in the following areas:

WE BELIEVE IN THE IMPORTANCE OF DEMONSTRATING CIVILITY TO PATIENTS, THEIR FAMILIES, AND OUR FELLOW STAFF MEMBERS.
Showing civility is the most significant contribution staff members can make to creating and sustaining psychological safety in their environment. Attending to what others contribute and responding with consideration not only reduces anxiety but encourages creative thinking.

WE BELIEVE IN THE IMPORTANCE OF PROFESSIONAL GOVERNANCE WHERE STAFF IS EMPOWERED TO CONTRIBUTE NEW IDEAS TO THE UNIT AND RESPECT THE VALUES AND BELIEFS OF OTHERS.
Contrasting ideas and views are a significant source of creativity. It is essential for team members to learn to be tolerant of other viewpoints.

The agreement should not be a mandatory value but agreeing to disagree respectfully should be. No one person is as smart as all of us.

WE BELIEVE THAT THE BEST PERFORMING TEAMS SUPPORT ONE ANOTHER AND RECOGNIZE THE VALUE OF COLLABORATION AND EXCELLENT COMMUNICATION.
Using supportive language towards others should be an expectation. Open hostility, anger and a failure to treat people with courtesy and respect will not be tolerated. Humor does not excuse a put-down nor does it make one palatable. People don't like it.

WE BELIEVE IN THE IMPORTANCE OF CREATING A SAFE ENVIRONMENT FOR PATIENTS, VISITORS AND STAFF.
To achieve both physical and psychological safety in an environment, staff need to feel comfortable and safe when reporting unsafe practices.

Maria knew that building an environment with psychological safety would take time. She also understood that feeling safe at work can increase the nurse's energy, enthusiasm, and zest for life.

ACCEPTING PERSONAL ACCOUNTABILITY FOR MISTAKES

Refusing to accept personal accountability in leadership leads to mistrust. Blaming others for work that you are ultimately responsible for can easily become a habit. When you become a leader, the buck stops with you. Contrary to what you might think, blaming others will not preserve your self-esteem because it comes at a high cost.

Jake learned this lesson the hard way. As manager of the operating room, he had accountability for ensuring that the cases were scheduled and that adjustments were made with changing patient priorities. Several surgeons went to his chief nursing officer (CNO) to complain about room rescheduling and a lack of communication regarding procedure time changes. They cited specific examples. The CNO called Jake in to discuss the problem. Instead of simply acknowledging what happened and apologizing for the lack of communication, Jake blamed his administrative assistant for failing to keep him on track with calls he needed to make to the surgeons. Jake's CNO became uneasy as he complained about the lack of organizational skills of his staff member. Jake's CNO told him she was disappointed in his response. She reminded him that leaders should never blame others for work that they are ultimately accountable to complete. It called into question his integrity as a leader and could damage staff trust in him.

Jake was ashamed at being confronted with his behavior and acknowledged it was a great coaching moment for him. His CNO helped him to gain perspective on behavior that would have ultimately damaged his effectiveness as a leader. Even if his assistant had made an error, it was his responsibility to coach her. When you commit as a leader and do not engage in the "blame game," then respect for you will skyrocket, others will follow you, and you will feel good about yourself. It often takes more courage to admit the truth. Ultimately, if you want staff to be professionally accountable for their work, you need to role model this behavior in your leadership practice. Professional accountability is also essential to be an authentic nurse leader.

AUTHENTICITY IN LEADERSHIP

When we think about an authentic leader, we look at someone who is true to himself or herself, someone who is honest and open, and someone who believes in his or her abilities. An authentic person does not hide anything from others and lives with integrity. Becoming an authentic leader is not a destination but rather a lifelong journey that is essential for successful nursing leadership. The American Association of Critical Care

Nurses included authentic leadership as one of the six standards necessary to establish and sustain a healthy work environment. [16] Components of authentic leadership include feeling a passion for the purpose of what you do as a leader, practicing solid values, leading with a heart, establishing enduring relationships and demonstrating self-discipline. There are some naturally authentic leaders, but most leaders need to work with intention to be authentic. Key steps include:

1. **COMMIT TO A PERSONAL JOURNEY TO BECOME MORE AUTHENTIC IN YOUR LEADERSHIP BY TAKING THE FOLLOWING ACTIONS:** [17]

   - Read books about authenticity in leadership.
   - Complete a self-assessment of personal strengths and identify your shadow side.
   - Develop the art of listening and self-reflection.
   - Insert humor into every aspect of life.
   - Commit to a philosophy of life-long learning.
   - Participate in leadership development opportunities.

2. **SEEK FEEDBACK FROM THOSE YOU LEAD.**
   Authentic leadership is not something that you declare is your leadership style. Your authenticity as a leader can only be validated by those that you lead. You must be willing to ask for and receive feedback openly. As you look to improve aspects of your leadership, a public declaration to your followers about a desire to grow can be very powerful.

3. **FIND A MENTOR WHO IS AN AUTHENTIC NURSE LEADER.**
   No one can be authentic by imitating another person but we can learn from their experiences. If you know a nurse leader that you admire for their authenticity, they can serve as a mentor for you on

your own journey. Life stories play a significant role in how great leaders become authentic.

4. HAVE A STRONG CONNECTION BETWEEN YOUR VALUES AND YOUR ACTIONS.

Authentic leaders clearly define which of their values cannot be violated regardless of the situation, and which values are desirable but not mandatory. Think carefully in advance how you will handle situations where your ethical boundaries and values conflict with the decisions you are asked to make. Your followers will carefully watch whether your values match your leadership actions.

5. WORK HARD TO BUILD RELATIONSHIPS AND ESTABLISH TRUST.

It is difficult to be perceived as authentic if you can't establish relationships with other people. If you are introverted, this may mean moving outside your comfort zone and being visible and approachable. Staff will want to know that you are connected to them and their work. They will also want to see that you can be trusted.

BE TRANSPARENT IN YOUR LEADERSHIP

In today's turbulent healthcare environment, many nurses complain that they have grown tired of working in settings where there is little transparency in decision making and that they often cannot trust their leaders to provide them with accurate information. The Gallup organization which has studied tens of thousands of employees over the past 30 years consistently finds that what staff value most in their leaders are the qualities of trust, compassion, hope and the ability to provide them with stable environments. [18]

Being transparent as a leader can be a powerful thing. Open leadership is the key to fostering a culture of trust between leaders and their employees. Nurses who are kept in the loop and understand their role in the overarching purpose and goals of their organization are more likely to put their trust in their employer. Your staff does not expect you to have all the answers but does want the truth. This may mean sometimes having to say that there are certain things that you cannot discuss at this time but will as soon as it is OK to share them. Staff wants you to be humble and even vulnerable.

From the perspective of leadership coaching, there are five good reasons to be transparent: [19]

1. **Problems can be solved faster** – Nursing staff often have remarkably good suggestions to solve problems if you have been transparent and they know they have all the information.

2. **Teams are built faster** – In a culture of trust and transparency, the stages of team development can move more quickly.

3. **Relationships grow more authentically** – Transparency allows coaching relationships to mature faster, as openness can potentially avoid misunderstandings that can fuel unnecessary tension.

4. **Staff promotes trust in their leader** – When leaders are transparent, people can be much more objective in evaluating the pros and cons of their leader. Through transparency especially in difficult situations, you strengthen your leadership as people begin to trust you as a person and thus respect you more as a leader. They will also share that trust in you with colleagues.

5. **Higher levels of performance emerge** – Nurses feel much better about their work when they think that they are in the know about what is happening in their organization – the good, the bad and the ugly. It is energizing to feel like you are part of a cohesive team.

Unfortunately, there is a lack of transparency that still exists among leaders in many healthcare workplaces. The irony is that these leaders lose in the long-run because performance on their teams will never reach the levels that could happen in a culture of transparency.

REMEMBER

✓ Trust is the foundation of a coaching relationship with staff.
✓ On a team with a culture of psychological safety, the leader encourages open discussion of tough issues.
✓ The key qualities that staff value most in their leaders are trust, compassion, hope and the ability to provide them with stable environments.
✓ Transparent leadership is key to fostering a culture of trust between leaders and their employees.

CHAPTER 4

ADOPT A TRANSFORMATIONAL LEADER STYLE

New leaders often struggle with what type of leader they want to be and what style of leadership is most effective. There is strong evidence that the most successful form of leadership in today's nursing environments is transformational leadership. It has been identified as a critical ingredient in the ANCC Magnet model because it has been shown to create environments that attract and retain nurses. [20] It is a leadership style that is a good fit for the nurse leader coach model.

First proposed in the mid-1970s, transformational leadership is described as occurring when "two or more persons engage with others in such a way that the leader and followers raise one another to high levels of motivation and morality." [21] At the time, this thinking was revolutionary and differed significantly from earlier leadership theories because it proposed that meeting the needs of followers was vital to achieving high work performance. In nursing, this was a significant change in thinking about leadership approaches. Like coaching, transformational leadership depends on a high level of engagement between the leader and followers. Traditionally, nursing leaders have used management styles ranging from an autocratic style, in which engagement goes in only one direction, to a "hands-off" or laissez-faire style, in which the manager is nearly disengaged.

BUILDING BLOCKS OF TRANSFORMATIONAL LEADERSHIP

Transformational leaders use the following four elements when leading others (Figure 4-1). [21]

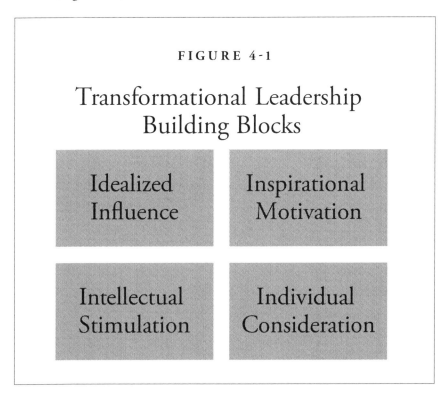

FIGURE 4-1

Transformational Leadership Building Blocks

Idealized Influence

Inspirational Motivation

Intellectual Stimulation

Individual Consideration

Idealized influence sometimes also called charisma, describes a leader's ability to inspire high standards and serve as a role model for outstanding professional practice. Such a leader gains the trust and respect of the staff.

Inspirational motivation refers to the leader's ability to communicate a vision that staff can understand and want to be a part of. For example, a nurse leader with a transformational style would find creative ways to inspire a team with a vision for the future. These could include meetings, Facebook postings, group texts, Twitter messages or using staff emails to communicate goals.

Intellectual stimulation is provided by a leader who asks for and values staff input, who challenges followers to develop creative and innovative solutions and who continually seeks ways to provide growth and development opportunities. A climate in which intellectual stimulation is supported prompts staff to challenge assumptions, to reframe problems and to look at new ways of doing things. For example, a transformational leader would provide time for nurses to learn about new evidence-based practice findings in patient care. Leaders who support intellectual stimulation find ways to encourage nurses to voice their ideas about improving patient care and pave the way for innovations to be tested and incorporated into the nursing culture.

Individualized consideration refers to the commitment of the leader to coaching, and mentoring and the leader's awareness of and concern for the needs of nursing staff. A transformational leader knows individual staff member's career aspirations and is often in a position to guide individuals to invaluable mentoring opportunities.

Nurse leaders who use transformational leadership principles create a climate in which nurses have a greater commitment to their organizations and high levels of morale, job satisfaction, and work performance. Transformational leadership, the preferred leadership style of Magnet hospitals, has been shown to motivate nurses to perform beyond expectations. Nurses by their nature are visionary, passionate, committed people who have innovative ideas about how to transform healthcare. Nurse leader coaches with a transformational leadership style can use this source of nursing knowledge to move nursing and patient care in a positive direction for the future.

STRATEGIES TO BECOME A TRANSFORMATIONAL LEADER

Like many new leaders, Mark was thrilled at the opportunity to lead others but also scared about whether he could be successful. He had assumed a director role in an ambulatory care center. The previous leader was well liked by staff but had not fostered their independence. Mark had concerns about how much they depended on the leader to set direction and make all decisions on the unit. He was determined to become a leader coach and needed to reset the leadership direction of the unit.

Mark had read about transformational leadership in his graduate program and decided he wanted to adopt that style of leadership. Most of what he learned seemed theoretical and he was not sure where to even begin or what to do to achieve his goal. He consulted his mentor who recommended the following four steps:

1. **PERSONALIZE YOUR MANAGEMENT STYLE**
   Transformational leaders learn about each individual staff member and when possible, give personal consideration. Staff members have

different personalities, needs, and skills and these should be honored. This is why having a one to one conversation with each staff member in the first 100 days in a leadership role is critical.

2. Encourage creativity

Transformational leaders foster innovation and creativity by challenging assumptions about what can and cannot be done. When staff take risks to improve care but make a mistake, be supportive of the risk-taking if you need to take corrective action. As a leader, focus on removing barriers to change and approach problems as learning opportunities. Ask staff to push back and challenge you on your ideas. In Mark's situation, this could be challenging initially because the team has become so dependent on their leader for guidance.

3. Guide, motivate and inspire

Transformational leaders have a positive mindset and exude motivation. Set a vision, strategy, and goals for a unit that are congruent with your health system but also motivational. Always connect the work of your unit staff to a greater purpose by keeping it patient-centered. Celebrate successes with enthusiasm. Show confidence in the ideas of your staff.

4. Be a role model

As a leader, you are always being watched. Your behavior will have more significant impact than words. Transformational leaders understand that they must walk the talk. Act with integrity and ethical standards; with both your behaviors and your words. Your team will take note of what you do and use it as a template for how they act and behave. It happens automatically and subconsciously, whether the behavior is positive or negative—people will follow your example.

Mark wondered how he would know if he was a transformational leader. This is an excellent question to ask. The interesting thing about transformational leadership is that it is your followers who will define what your leadership style is not you. Many leaders describe themselves as transformational, but their staff would disagree. Without evidence, declaring oneself to be transformational is a personal opinion that may or may not be verified by those who work for the leader. Developing transformational leadership skills requires that nurse leaders be honest and reflective about their current practices.

Fortunately, there are good questions that you can ask yourself to be sure that you are on the right track. Dr. Ronald Riggio, an expert in leadership development, advises leaders to ask themselves the following key questions (or ask their staff) to determine whether they demonstrate transformational leader qualities: (Agree or Disagree) [22]

1. I would never require a follower to do something that I would not do myself.
2. My followers would say they know what I stand for.
3. Inspiring others has always come easily to me.
4. My followers would say that I am attentive to their needs and concerns.
5. My followers have told me that my enthusiasm and positive energy is infectious.
6. Even though I could easily do a task myself, I delegate it to expand my follower's skills.
7. Team creativity and innovation are the keys to success.
8. I encourage my followers to question their most basic way of thinking.

DON'T BE AN IDEA KILLER

Transformational leaders encourage creativity and new ways of doing things even if they have been tried before and did not work. To promote innovation, you cannot be an idea killer. This was Kathryn's problem. With over ten years of management experience, Kathryn was proud of her leadership track record. She was therefore surprised by comments from her Millennial staff on a recent employee satisfaction survey that indicated she was an idea killer. She had not perceived herself this way but realized on reflection that she did shoot down many new ideas with phrases such as: "Well that's a great idea, but we can't do that here, or We've never done anything like that."

Kathrynn's situation is a good reminder for those who have been in leadership for years to consider whether they are idea killers. Start by asking yourself the following questions:

1. **DO YOU BELIEVE THAT YOUR EXPERIENCE ENTITLES YOU TO JUDGE WHETHER AN IDEA IS A GOOD ONE OR A BAD ONE?**
   As a leader, you naturally have preferred ways of getting things done or solving problems, but your way may not be the only way. It is important to give staff the accountability and responsibility to make decisions and take action without the need to seek your approval. Ask yourself whether you feel threatened when presented with new information.

2. **DO YOU BELIEVE THAT FAILURE IS NOT AN OPTION?**
   Much can be learned from failure. Some initiatives don't work but we have to be willing to let others try. As a nurse leader, you quickly learn that not every staff member on your team will be successful. Allowing someone to fail and maintain their dignity can be the absolutely right thing to do in leadership.

3. **DO YOU REGULARLY QUESTION YOUR ASSUMPTIONS?**

   Killing new ideas could mean that you are failing to question your own assumptions which may not be correct. What if you are wrong? What if circumstances have changed? What if there is new evidence to support that something should be done a different way?

4. **DO YOU RESPOND TO NEW IDEAS BY SAYING "THAT CAN'T BE DONE"?**

   There is no greater idea killer than the phrase "that can't be done." Some leaders quickly respond to suggestions with this phrase. Even when the suggestion seems outside the bounds of what can be done in an organization – a better response would be that you are not sure it is doable, but together you should investigate the possibilities.

As we move forward with health care reform, it is likely that some of our basic assumptions about nursing and healthcare will be tested. The key to effective nursing leadership may be "unlearning" some of what we may have always believed. It will also require a willingness to set aside some of our sacred cows. This means listening to and being open to new and different ideas and carefully monitoring the language that we use.

SHIFTING FROM "BUT" TO "YES, AND"

The word **but** is a conversation killer. It sends the message that whoever brings up the new idea is being denied the opportunity to go further. Often it is said by someone who enjoys the role of devil's advocate and wants to look smart and discerning. A slight shift in language to "yes, and" can become a powerful tool for collaboration, negotiation, and effective communication. It makes people feel valued, supported and heard.

The origins of "yes, and" started in the world of improvisation with Second City in Chicago. Comic improvisation is an art form where 5-6 actors arrive on the stage with no scripts, props or costumes. [23] The show has a general topic but the actors have to create the show at the moment without knowing where it is headed. It works because of the "yes, and" approach. One actor starts the conversation with a topic such as "Last night I had dinner with my mother," and a second actor will jump in with "Yes, and what did she make for dinner?" The conversation builds on this topic with a yes, and approach resulting in what looks like a one-act play by continually accepting what is being contributed onstage.

The "yes, and" approach can be powerful for leaders. You send the message that you are open and want to give every idea an opportunity to be discussed. You don't negate it, belittle it or disagree with it. "Yes, and" may not be right for every situation, but try it in your leadership practice. So, the next time you are inclined to say something like *but we don't have the budget,* try instead to frame it differently, *Yes, and let's figure out whether we can make this budget neutral.* You may be surprised how that changes the conversation and how others will view your leadership as transformational.

LIGHT FIRES – DON'T EXTINGUISH FLAMES

The inventor and philosopher Albert Schweitzer once said "*in everyone's life, at some time, our inner fire goes out. It is then burst into flames by an encounter with another human being. We should all be thankful to those people who rekindle our inner spirit*". [24] Transformational nurse leaders recognize that as a coach, they can be fire starters and can rekindle the fire within where it has been extinguished. This involves giving individualized consideration to staff.

Jason saw this in his leadership practice. One of his senior nurses was disengaged from her work, and he heard rumors that she might quit. He took the time to have a coaching session with her and learned that she was having a challenging time at home since her youngest child had left for college. She no longer felt valued. Jason wisely recognized that this nurse needed to nurture others. She was his strongest preceptor. He spoke with his supervisor about giving her a special project to revise their unit orientation. Part of the work would involve attending a professional conference about best practices in new graduate orientation. This simple act of reaching out, having a life coaching conversation and giving this nurse a stretch assignment had a remarkable impact and relit her passion for her work. Are you a fire starter or a flame extinguisher? The following are some key questions you can ask yourself:

Fire Starter Behaviors

- Do you show compassion when a staff member has difficult challenges?
- Do you look for the strengths of your staff members and not focus on weaknesses?
- Do you individualize your leadership to meet the needs of your staff?
- Do you show encouragement for innovation?
- Do you give staff stretch assignments to help them grow?
- Do you celebrate staff achievements?
- Do you encourage a culture of learning?
- Do you communicate and communicate and communicate?
- Do you give hope during challenging times?
- Do you listen with your eyes, your ears and your heart?
- Do you show appreciation to others?
- Do you look for opportunities to help others shine?
- Do you give credit to others for their work?
- Are you passionate and enthusiastic?

Fire Extinguisher Behaviors

- Do you blame others for your leadership failures?
- Are you threatened by high performing staff?
- Do you focus on deficits instead of strengths?
- Do you use words like "no", "but" or "however" in conversations about new ideas?
- Do you fail to listen to viewpoints that are different from your own?
- Do you hesitate to acknowledge when you are wrong?
- Are you pessimistic during times of instability?
- Do you believe the staff is lucky to have a job?
- Do you feel the staff should leave their personal problems at home?
- Do you fail to give others second chances?
- Do you withhold information that would be valuable to helping others?
- Do you lack passion for your work?
- Are you unapproachable?
- Do fail to respond to messages?
- Do you spend most of your day in your office?

Firestarter leaders love to coach, mentor and develop others. They look for the best in the individual and leave a rich legacy when their work is done. By contrast, fire extinguishers cause stress, burnout, and disengagement in staff who work with and for them. Which one would you rather work for?

REMEMBER

- ✓ There is strong evidence that the most successful style of leadership in today's nursing environments is transformational leadership.
- ✓ Transformational leadership, the preferred leadership style of Magnet hospitals, has been shown to motivate nurses to perform beyond expectations.
- ✓ To encourage innovation, you cannot be an idea killer.
- ✓ The word **but** is a conversation killer. It sends the message that whoever brings up the new idea is being denied the opportunity to go further.

CHAPTER 5

ESTABLISH A CULTURE OF LEARNING

Effective nurse leader coaches establish a culture of learning in their units. When you value learning, you recognize that it is the path to mastery. You also set clear expectations that professional growth is a critical part of nursing practice. There are five key ways that you can build a culture of learning in your unit.

1. VALUE EVIDENCE-BASED PRACTICE

Evidence-based nursing practice is widely recognized as being essential to achieving the best patient outcomes. Yet, the research indicates that most nurse leaders don't use evidence-based leadership practices. In a survey of over 1000 ANA members, nurses were asked whether their managers consistently make evidence-based decisions. On a Likert scale of 1 (strongly disagree) to 5 (strongly agree), the mean for Magnet hospitals was 3.6, and for non-Magnet, it was 3.1.[25] These are disappointing findings. To be successful as a nurse leader, you need to continually challenge your assumptions and be willing to look at the best scientific evidence available to guide your decision making. This includes not only clinical practice but also leadership practice.

2. Look for the Lessons Learned in Every Situation

Reflective practice is part of a culture of learning. When there is a challenging situation or if there has been an adverse patient outcome, there are always lessons learned. Leaders should frequently ask the staff, *"What are the lessons learned here and how could we do it differently the next time?"*

3. Celebrate Staff Learning and Educational Achievements

It is often said in leadership that what gets rewarded is what is valued. To establish a culture of learning, educational achievements must be valued. Staff should be celebrated when they complete a degree or achieve certification. You want to send a powerful message that these achievements matter.

4. Volunteer for Innovative Projects and Pilot Programs

I recently visited a dedicated education unit (DEU) in a hospital that was designed to both improve new graduate orientation and medical-surgical staff retention. I was curious about how the specific units were selected to participate in the project. Not surprisingly, I heard that it was the nurse manager on this unit that stepped forward and said that they wanted to be involved. Leaders who want to establish a culture of learning know that being part of innovative projects and pilot programs can be very energizing to staff. It sets your team apart as a group that is willing to change and innovate.

5. MODEL THE WAY AS A LEADER

As a leader, staff will watch to see if you walk the talk. Your personal feelings about whether you value learning will show in how you discuss issues such as knowledge, information, and change. Ask yourself the following questions:

- Have you continued your education?
- Do you stay updated on the latest trends?
- Are you curious and open to new information?
- Are you certified?
- Do you allow staff to challenge a process that may need to be changed?
- Do you prefer to hire staff who have completed a BSN or MSN?
- Do you do a periodic assessment of your staff's learning needs?
- Do you ask for learning-related goals for the upcoming year when you do staff evaluations?
- Do you have regular unit/department education?

Building a culture of learning on your unit or in your department is an ongoing journey. There is strong evidence to indicate that the payoffs can be significant, with better patient outcomes and a more highly committed staff.

PROMOTING A GROWTH VERSUS A FIXED MINDSET

Sometimes highly committed nurse leader coaches may encounter resistance to establishing a culture of learning. This happened to David when he assumed a manager role in a labor and delivery unit. The CNO who had hired him indicated that she had concerns that practices were outdated on the unit, and not based on the most recent evidence for OB care. David seemed like the right candidate to build a learning culture on the unit. He was certified in his specialty area, had gone back for a graduate degree and was active in his professional specialty association. He was surprised to learn that some of his staff did not share his enthusiasm for professional growth. In his initial meetings with staff, he indicated his desire to be a leader coach and help staff to grow and develop professionally. Several nurses told David that they were there to put in their 12 hours and did not want to be coached to grow in their careers. Their previous manager had not pushed them professionally and some staff seemed annoyed that David was setting this as an expectation. This reaction was hard for David to understand because he himself was a lifelong learner.

Part of David's leadership challenge in this situation is helping staff move from a "fixed mindset" to a "growth mindset." Dr. Carol Dweck, a researcher and professor at Stanford University, has been a pioneer in studying how transformative a growth mindset can be for individuals and overall well-being. A *mindset*, according to Dweck, is a self-perception or "self-theory" that people hold about themselves.[26] Mindsets can either be growth oriented or fixed (Figure 5-1). In a growth mindset, people believe that their skills and abilities can be developed through dedication and hard work—brains and talent are just the starting point. This view creates a love of learning and a resilience that is essential for great accomplishment. In contrast, when the staff has a fixed mindset, they may believe that they can no longer grow professionally. They are less willing to adopt new changes or open themselves to new experiences because it could be threatening.

When you have a growth mindset, you believe that you can and will learn and achieve. A growth mindset results in a powerful belief that anyone can accomplish more if they decide to learn, work, and develop the necessary skills. With a growth mindset, when you fail, you'll figure out what went wrong and work on making sure it doesn't happen next time. You don't write yourself off and are willing to step outside your comfort zone.

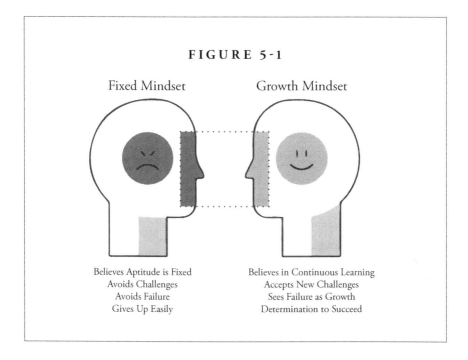

FIGURE 5-1

Fixed Mindset   Growth Mindset

Believes Aptitude is Fixed   Believes in Continuous Learning
Avoids Challenges   Accepts New Challenges
Avoids Failure   Sees Failure as Growth
Gives Up Easily   Determination to Succeed

Nurse leader coaches can be instrumental in helping staff move from a fixed to a growth mindset. Fixed mindsets often evolve when staff are insecure or have had failures in their past experience. Over time, David can work with his staff using the following strategies:

- Create a new compelling belief about what is possible and how individuals can contribute.
- Reframe failures that happen on the unit as growth experiences.
- Focus and help staff to learn more about their strengths.
- Introduce learning in a fun and non-threatening way.
- Reinforce successes that the individual has in the face of challenges.
- Reward achievements even the small steps.

Confront Deviations from Acceptable Practice

New managers like David sometimes find clinical practices in their unit that are clear deviations from acceptable practice and organizational policies. As a leader coach, it is essential to have the courage to call out deviant practices. The normalization of deviance is defined as a gradual process in which an unacceptable practice or standards become acceptable. As the deviant behavior is repeated without catastrophic results, it becomes the social norm for the unit culture. With medical errors now the 3rd leading cause of death in hospitals today, it is very problematic when small incremental deviances are tolerated and become behavioral norms.

Factors Leading to Deviance

Interestingly it has been found in research that deviant behavior is more likely to occur in experienced versus inexperienced staff. As nurses become more confident about their judgment, they are more likely to believe that they can bend the rules slightly if needed. John Banja cites seven factors that lead to the normalization of deviant behavior in healthcare environments: [27]

1. Staff believes that rules are stupid and inefficient, developed by those who are not in the trenches of care.
2. Staff knowledge is imperfect and uneven, and some staff may not even know the reasons for the practice and procedure.
3. New technologies can disrupt ingrained practice patterns, impose new learning demands, or force system operators to devise novel responses or accommodations to new work challenges.
4. Staff believes that it is OK to break a rule for the good of the patient.

5. Staff believes that rules don't apply to them; they have experience and can be trusted.

6. Staff fears speaking up when deviant behavior is observed.

7. There is leadership awareness of deviant behavior or systems problems, but there is a failure to bring it up the chain of command.

Challenging Deviant Behavior

To counter deviant behavior, nurse leader coaches must have a fundamental commitment to patient safety and this must be evident to staff. Leaders should be acutely vigilant about deviant behaviors and practices and be ready to take aggressive steps to halt their occurrence before they achieve normalization. Deviations or rule violations are rarely motivated by malice or greed but often result from nursing staff feeling intense performance pressures.

The best time for the nurse leader coach to intervene in correcting a deviant practice is early rather than later on when righting the now-normalized deviation can be much more challenging. When you counsel staff for errors—watch for the statement *"staff on this unit do this all the time—I am not the only one."* It could be a defensive response but it might also indicate the normalization of a deviant behavior. Your goal should be to create a culture of learning where some practice deviations could occur, but where they receive swift attention. Staff also need to be taught to feel comfortable in speaking up when they see deviant behaviors.

Recognize Failure is Part of Learning

Nurse leader coaches recognize that failure is part of learning. As manager of an invasive cardiology department, Christine needed to coach her staff about a serious medication error that had resulted in a patient injury. In the root cause analysis done by the quality department, it was determined that a contributing factor to the error was staff competency in caring for the patient. The error involved a relatively new graduate nurse who received an inadequate orientation to her role responsibilities and lacked expected competencies.

Christine recognized that with the retirement of many of her seasoned staff, the majority of her nurses now had less than two years of experience. As an outcome of the staffing mix changes, the supervision and orientation of the new graduate was not adequate. The nurse involved in the error had been assigned to care for a patient whose care was too complex given her level of competency. The new graduate was devastated by the mistake and needed coaching to regain her resiliency. Christine realized that it was a lesson learned for both her and her staff. She accepted full accountability and responsibility to work on the problems that led to the error. In her coaching, Christine recognized that young nurses fear failure and expect that they will never make errors. She knew this is unrealistic and part of her coaching was to show the young nurse how this error could be a transformative step in her career.

While failure is part of the nursing experience, we don't often either write about it or publicly discuss it. We celebrate our successes and focus on what is working in organizations. Yet, reflection is vital after failure to learn and grow from the experience. Leaders should avoid the blame game when there is a failure. We often find that errors are a result of a wider systems problem. Some key questions to ask include:

- What happened and why?
- What vital signs did I miss leading up to the failure?
- What were the consequences of what happened here?
- What did I learn as a nurse from this situation?
- How will I apply any lessons learned in the future?

Our failures can be some of our best teachers if we pay attention and learn from them. Managing failure well is key to establishing a culture of learning.

Value Certification to Promote Professional Growth

Nurse leader coaches recognize the importance of certification to get their staff more engaged in their work and professional growth. There is strong evidence that patient outcomes improve when more nurses working in a unit are certified.[28] Nurses who are certified are better informed about new changes in practice and more likely to provide evidence-based care. They are also far more likely to "own their practice" and to do the right thing because they expect it of themselves. Engagement scores among certified nurses are higher because they have a genuine interest in learning more about their specialty areas. This power over practice and having a strong purpose is also known to promote staff resiliency.

Given the many benefits that nurses experience by becoming certified, Jason was surprised that only 20% of his emergency department staff had sought certification. His professional association had recently released a whitepaper outlining compelling reasons for ED nurses to achieve and maintain certification.[29] Nurses with certification were found to have higher self-efficacy, more knowledge about emergency care trends and greater career success.

When asked why they had not become certified, nurses in his department cited the cost, time, lack of organizational incentives, limited perceived value and a fear of failure. While Jason understood that his safety net hospital had few resources to provide funding for certification, he also realized that we define what is important to us by how we spend our time and money. As a leader coach, he was determined to coach his nurses about the importance of certification. He recognized that he needed to walk the talk so he became certified as a first step. He worked with his ED educator to provide a review course and became a cheerleader for the certification initiative. Jason recognized that the possibility of failure was a significant concern and he worked on building the confidence level of his staff. He made certification achievement a key value in the culture. He would not accept excuses for not being certified because he believed given the evidence, that there was too much at stake not to make it an expectation.

REMEMBER

✓ Effective nurse leader coaches establish a culture of learning in their units.

✓ Evidence-based nursing practice is widely recognized as being essential to achieving the best patient outcomes.

✓ As a leader coach, it is essential to have the courage to call out deviant practices.

✓ Our failures can be some of our best teachers if we pay attention and learn from them.

✓ Nurse leader coaches recognize the importance of certification to get their staff more engaged in their work and professional growth.

CHAPTER 6

CREATE TIME TO COACH

Many managers will say that they don't have the time to coach. If you reframe your thinking about the importance of coaching from a "nice to do" to a "must do," time will not be a problem. In today's job market, there is fierce competition for good talent. If you commit yourself to be a leader coach, you could considerably decrease the time that you spend recruiting new staff. Sally learned this the hard way when she took her first leadership role on a medical-surgical unit. Her mentor had recommended that she have a short one-on-one conversation with each staff member during her first 100 days in the position. These meetings were intended to learn more about the staff member, establish trust and set the foundation for a coaching relationship. Sally had met with less than half of her staff. Six months into her new role, her unit had a 20% turnover rate and her Gallup Q12 engagement scores were low. Much of her time is now consumed with the recruitment and orientation of new staff.

For many nurse leaders, the toughest part of a leadership role is organizing and putting boundaries around their work. When nurses like Sally begin in leadership, they often find themselves spending too much time in their comfort zone which is usually in clinical patient care. When you move into administration, your role shifts from caring for patients to caring for staff. Effective nurse leader coaches recognize that coaching conversations can be short, but these interactions must be intentional.

Learning to carve out time to do this and your administrative responsibilities can be challenging. It is not uncommon to hear that nurse leaders work 10-12 hours each day, and then continue to answer texts and emails on the weekend. While this level of commitment may seem commendable, it can lead to stress and burnout. The problem with not having boundaries in leadership work is that the pace of work can become unsustainable. Leaders may feel that the only way out to regain control is to leave their position. There is a culture in some settings where working long hours and not taking breaks is a badge of honor. Nurses look to their leaders to role model good work-life balance but too often they see quite the opposite.

SETTING LEADERSHIP BOUNDARIES

Boundaries serve many functions in helping us to regain control of our lives.[30] They help to protect us, to clarify what is our responsibility and what is another's, to preserve our physical and emotional energy, to stay focused on ourselves, to live our values and standards, and to identify our limits. The following steps can help you to set better boundaries:

Step 1 – Identify your limits – We are often our own worst enemies when it comes to working and can have challenges saying no. Set limits on how many meetings you attend, how long you stay at work each day and hours you can be contacted at home. This guides you to know when you are stepping over lines and moving into destructive patterns. Limits are a very individual thing and may vary considerably among leaders. A nurse leader with young children is usually at a different life stage with more demands on their time than a leader with grown children.

Step 2 – Pay attention to your feelings – Feelings are an important gauge of whether we have moved into overdrive with our work. Pay close attention when you feel discomfort, resentment or guilt. These feelings are often signs that a boundary issue may be present. If you have these feelings repeatedly, then it is time to restructure your boundaries.

Step 3 – Give yourself permission to set boundaries – Nurse leaders often feel they should be able to cope with a situation and say yes because that is what they are expected to do. You may question whether you even have the right or deserve to set boundaries in the first place. When these doubts occur, reaffirm to yourself that you do indeed have this right, so give yourself permission set limits, and work to preserve them.

Step 4 – Consider your environment – Work environment can play a crucial role in how comfortable leaders are in setting boundaries. Your environment can either support your setting boundaries or present obstacles to boundary setting which makes it more challenging. Nurse executives play such a key role in making it OK (even demanding it) for their leaders to set boundaries.

DETERMINE WHAT IS ESSENTIAL

We live in a noisy world. This is especially true in healthcare where there are significant changes almost daily that impact our work. The pace of change has taken a toll on even the most adaptive nurse leaders.

Leaders find themselves spread so thin in their work that finding a sense of real accomplishment becomes challenging and finding time to coach is impossible. Many nurse leaders describe the problem as one of time management. But will there ever be enough time to accomplish all that we want to? Greg McKeown, an expert on time management, counters that NO there will never be enough time if we are not disciplined in our approach to concentrate on what matters most. [31]

Essentialism is training our brain to focus on what is essential in our work. It means saying no to projects, meetings, commitments, and activities that don't advance the quality of our work. It is committing to and being willing, as McKeown describes it, to "go big" for the few vital activities that will have the most impact such as coaching. [31] It involves making the trade-offs that come with not involving yourself and a recognition that to become really good at our work, we need to focus on what matters most. You then begin living by design and not by default. Steve Jobs, the founder of Apple, often credited his success with being able to say yes to what really mattered and no to a thousand other things.

Becoming an essentialist is not easy if you have a hard time saying no. You may feel like you are disappointing people by saying no, yet in the long-term essentialist leaders become highly respected for their discipline and focus. They recognize that more effort does not necessarily yield better results. You will find that you become a better leader when you can say no to opportunities that are not essential to your work. Here are ten key steps: to developing the essentialist habit:

1. Decide what in your work has the highest impact and yields the most significant results such as coaching.
2. Create space/time in your life to concentrate and think.
3. Stop worrying about FOMO or a fear of missing out and develop a willingness to accept decisions made without you in areas that don't have a significant impact on your work.

4. Get enough sleep to enable you to be most effective.

5. Vigorously evaluate your need for participation in every event or a new project, and rate the importance on a scale 0-100. If it is less than 90, it may be unessential. If it is not a clear yes, then it is probably a no.

6. Review all your current activities and priorities with the idea of eliminating the trivial many.

7. Say no gracefully, and separate the decision from the relationship.

8. Cut your losses quickly if something is not working.

9. Take time out to have fun.

10. View setting boundaries as a source of liberation.

CLARIFY EXPECTATIONS ABOUT MEETING ATTENDANCE

A significant frustration for many leaders is the number of meetings held in their organizations or health systems that they are expected to attend. Managing time is challenging for nurse leaders in today's environment. Many leaders struggle with trying to be everywhere. It is important early in your leadership tenure to gain clarity on which meetings are essential for you to attend personally and which ones are not. Some leaders believe that the only way they can stay in the loop in their organizations is to personally attend all the meetings that are scheduled. They have a fear of missing out (FOMO). While going to many meetings may make you feel important, it may not be the best allocation of your time. You need to learn to give yourself permission to decline meetings. Some other suggestions about meeting include the following:

1. Always ask for the agenda in advance and ask yourself whether you really need to be there. Perhaps the meeting could be attended

by another staff member or maybe you only need to be present for part of the meeting.

2. When you do attend – be present and engaged. Put away your smartphone. When we are frustrated at meetings, the easiest path is often just to disengage from what is being discussed. A second path is to endlessly complain that nothing is being accomplished even though we ourselves are not contributing any outcomes. Neither approach enhances our image as leaders.

3. Avoid being the one who convenes an unnecessary meeting. Determine whether there is there another way to reach a decision such as an email or a phone call.

Doing What Matters Most

Translating what matters most into action can be challenging. Jennifer experienced this in her first leadership role. She had good intentions at the beginning of each day but found herself working long hours with few things on her task list completed. Too often in our nursing leadership work, we create long task lists of goals that we want to accomplish. When we create these task lists, we can make the mistake of thinking that everything matters equally but the truth is that it doesn't. Success is sequential, not simultaneous. It's one step at a time.

Gary Keller, in *The One Thing: The Surprising Simple Truth Behind Extraordinary Results,* suggests that we focus on the one thing right now that will matter most.[32] This one thing may not be the one and the only thing on your to-do list, but it is the ONE THING right now. Keller is a firm believer in the Pareto principle or the 80/20 law of the vital few. This principle has research support. Using your efforts at work as an example, the law proposes that a minority (20%) of actions, inputs, and efforts leads to a majority of results, outputs or rewards. In other words, a small amount of effort in the right areas can lead to the greatest rewards. You need to look for an action that will lead to the domino effect. Trying to multitask and make many things happen at once is overrated in terms of effectiveness.

When thinking about what matters most, Jennifer decided that coaching her staff would have the biggest payback on her unit outcomes and staff satisfaction yet she was spending little time doing it. She decided to recommit to coaching by being intentional about planning three coaching conversations each day with staff, allowing for up to 15 minutes for each. Jennifer recognized that this did not have to be a huge commitment of her time. Instead, what mattered is that she was present in the conversation and asked good open-ended questions. These conversations could be recognizing good work, pointing out skills progression, discussing career goals or just asking questions related to the staff's well-being. Like most of us, Jennifer instinctively knew what matters most. It is taking the next step that becomes important, and that means going small for the fewer things that will have the most effect.

LEARN TO SAY NO

Your time is a limited commodity. This means that every time you make a commitment, it will leave less time for other activities. A reality of leadership is that the more successful we are, the less accessible we become. Brad learned this lesson. He was a natural people pleaser who had a hard time saying no in his leadership role. For a short time, his agreeableness served him well. Both his staff and his supervisors loved working with him. Later, he found himself overcommitted and not following through on promises he made to his staff and organization. He was losing trust each time he failed to deliver on a commitment or waited until the last minute to complete a request.

A leader can't be equally accessible to all people. This leaves you with the dilemma of who gets your time and who doesn't. You also need to decide when do they get it and how much time do, they get. Requests for your time are in a sense an affirmation that you are successful in your work. While this can be very flattering, you can also easily burn out from becoming overcommitted, as Brad did. Learning to say no to more requests can be one of the biggest favors you can do for both yourself and your staff. It helps to reduce your stress level and gives you time for what's important, like coaching.

When you say no to a new commitment, you are in fact honoring your existing obligations. You are also ensuring that you will be able to devote quality time to them. Having said this, it can be challenging to say no. You may worry that you are missing out on a great opportunity. It is important to remember that saying no may give you time for different opportunities that may be more important either personally or professionally. Here are some statements that you can use to say no in a positive way. [5]

> *I would love to be involved but I can't commit to this as I have other priorities.*
>
> *Now's is not a good time as I'm in the middle of something else. I may be able to do this at another time.*
>
> *I'm not the best person to help you with this. Why don't you try (offer a suggestion)?*
>
> *This sounds like an interesting opportunity, but no I can't do it.*

Saying no can be difficult but most of us have also found ourselves in situations where we said yes reluctantly, and later regretted our decision. Some people will be pushy so you need to learn to be firm but polite in your choices. Don't leave the door open for further negotiation. You may find yourself saying no to good things to focus on higher priorities.

Saying no may also allow you to try new things. If you have volunteered for five years to chair a heart walk, it may be time to give someone else the opportunity. It is important to recognize that your resources are finite to avoid the guilt trap. Saying no is about respecting and valuing your time and space. If done well, people may not be happy with your refusal but they will understand. You will find more time to be a leader coach.

REMEMBER

- ✓ Setting boundaries around your work is essential to stay balanced.
- ✓ There will never be enough time to accomplish everything so determine what is essential.
- ✓ Essentialism is recognizing you can do anything but not everything.
- ✓ When you learn to say no – you are honoring the obligations that you have already made.

References – Part 1

1. Mancino D. *National Student Nurses Association Survey Data* . AONE Conference. 2018.
2. Gallup Research. (2018). Transforming managers into coaches. Presentation Gallup Clifton Strengths Summit. 2018.
3. Bungay-Stanier M. *The Coaching Habit: Say, Less, Ask More + Change the Way You Lead Forever.* Toronto: Box of Crayons Press; 2016.
4. Wooden J, Carty J. *Coach Wooden's Pyramid of Success:* Ada, MO: Revell Publishers; 2009.
5. Whitemore J. *Coaching for Performance: The Principles and Practices of Coaching and Leadership 5th Edition.* London: Nicholas Brealey Publishers; 2017.
6. Bluepoint Leadership. *Top Ten Coaching Mistakes.;* 2016. Available at https://www.youtube.com/watch?v=MV0hAmtF1EA. Accessed July 1, 2018.
7. Kouzes JM, Posner BZ. *The Leadership Challenge 6th Edition.* Hoboken, NJ: John Wiley & Sons; 2017.
8. Drucker P. Managing yourself. *Harvard Business Review.* 2005; 83: 100-109.

9. Goldberg L. The structure of phenotypic personality traits". *American Psychologist.* 1993 48: 26–34

10. Goleman D. *Emotional Intelligence: Why It Can Matter More than IQ.* New York: Bantam Books; 2005.

11. Goldsmith M. *What Got You Here Won't Get You There: How Successful People Become Even More Successful.* New York: Hachette Books; 2007.

12. Roger D, Petrie N. *Work with stress: Building a resilient mindset for lasting success.* New York: McGraw-Hill; 2017.

13. Covey SR. *7 Habits of Highly Effective People.* New York: Free Press; 1989.

14. Horsager D. *The Trust Edge: How Top Leaders Gain Results Faster, Deeper Relationships and a Stronger Bottom Line.* New York: Free Press; 2012.

15. Edmondson A. *Building a Psychologically Safe Workplace;* 2014. Available at https://www.youtube.com/watch?v=LhoLuui9gX8 Accessed July 5th, 2018.

16. American Association of Critical Care Nurse. *AACN Standards for Building and Sustaining Healthy Work Environments.* https://www.aacn.org/nursing-excellence/standards/aacn-standards-for-establishing-and-sustaining-healthy-work-environments. Published 2005. Accessed July 7th, 2018.

17. Shirey, M. Authentic leaders creating healthy work environments for nursing practice. *American Journal of Critical Care. 2006;* 15: 256-267.

18. Gallup. *First Break all the Rules: What the World's Greatest Managers Do Differently.* New York: Gallup Press; 2016.

19. Lopis G. (September 10, 2012, Forbes Blog). Five things happen when a leader is transparent. Available at https://www.forbes.com/sites/glennllopis/2012/09/10/5-powerful-things-happen-when-a-leader-is-transparent/#6d6f782e4a3a. Accessed July 13th, 2018.

20. American Nursing Credentialing Center. The Magnet Model. Available at https://www.nursingworld.org/organizational-programs/magnet/magnet-model/ Accessed July 13th, 2018.

21. Burns JM. *Transforming Leadership.* New York: Grove Press; 2004.

22. Riggio RE. (March 24th, 2009 Psychology Today Blog). Are you a transformational leader? Available at https://www.psychologytoday.com/us/blog/cutting-edge-leadership/200903/are-you-transformational-leader Accessed July 13th, 2018.

23. Leonard K, Yorton T. Yes, And: How Improvisation Reverses "No, But" Thinking and Improves Creativity and Collaboration-Lessons from the Second City. New York: Harper Business; 2015.

24. Albert Schweitzer quotes. Available at https://www.goodreads.com/author/quotes/47146.Albert_Schweitzer. Accessed July 14th, 2018.

25. Melynk BM, Fineout-Overholt E, Gallagher-Ford L, Kaplan L. The state of evidence-based practice in US nurses: critical implications for nurse leaders and educators. *Journal Nursing Administration.* 2012; 42: 410-417.

26. Dweck CS. Mindset the New Psychology of Success. New York: Penguin Publishers; 2016.

27. Banja, J. The normalization of deviance in healthcare delivery. *Business Horizons.* 2010; 53:139 Available at http://www.ncbi.nlm.nih.gov/pmc/articles/PMC2821100/

28. American Association of Critical-Care Nurses [AACN]. (2015). Nurse certification benefits patients, employers and nurses. Available at https://www.aacn.org/certification/value-of-certification-resource-center/nurse-certification-benefits-patients-employers-and-nurses Accessed July 21st, 2018.

29. Board of Certification for Emergency Nursing. (2018). 5 compelling reasons to get (and keep) your emergency nursing specialty certification. Available at https://www.bcencertifications.org/Tools-Resources/BCEN-Whitepaper/BCEN-Whitepaper-Nurses Accessed July 21st, 2018.

30. Gionta DA, Guerra D. *From Stress to Centered: A Practical Guide for a Happier and Healthier You.* From Stressed to Centered; 2015.
31. McKeown G. *Essentialism: The Disciplined Pursuit of Less.* Australia: Currency Publishers; 2014.
32. Keller G. *The ONE Thing: The Surprising Simple Truth Behind Extraordinary Results.* Chicago: Bard Press; 2013.

DEVELOPING YOUR COACHING SKILLS

"Coaching should be a daily, informal act, not an occasional, formal "It's Coaching Time" event."

MICHAEL BUNGAY STANIER

CHAPTER 7

FOSTER STAFF ENGAGEMENT

A s we learned in Part 1 of the book, the path to becoming a successful nurse leader coach begins with building a strong foundation for coaching activities. In Part 2, we will look at some of the key skills needed to coach effectively. The ideal coaching situation is one in which staff is engaged in their work. Unfortunately, this is not always the case, and the initial efforts of the leader coach may need to focus on rebuilding engagement.

Data from a 2017 State of the American Workplace Report from the Gallup organization indicates that only 33% of US employees are engaged in their work, the others are either not engaged or actively disengaged. [1] These trends are consistent with national research conducted by the Nurse Advisory Board which indicates that only 32.8% of Registered Nurses are engaged in their work, and 7.4% are actively disengaged. [2] Statistically, professional nurses have lower work engagement and higher disengagement rates than other frontline staff in healthcare agencies.

This is troubling because nurses contribute substantially to the patient care experience and are also crucial in efforts to transform healthcare. When evaluating engagement, there are the following three levels:

- **Engaged** – employees who are loyal and committed to the organization. They are highly productive and more likely to stay in their roles.
- **Not Engaged** – these employees may be productive, but they are not psychologically connected to their organization. They are more likely to miss workdays and leave the organization.
- **Actively Disengaged** – these employees are physically present but psychologically absent. They are not only unhappy about their work situation but readily share this unhappiness with other professional colleagues.

Through their research, Gallup has found that staff engagement has a direct impact on the organization's bottom line and customer satisfaction. The good news is that leaders who are committed to coaching employees can make a significant difference in employee engagement. However, employee engagement is not a one size fits all strategy. Different staff members may need different engagement strategies, and that is where individualized coaching is vital.

Managers sometimes misunderstand staff engagement. It is not the same as staff satisfaction which generally measures perks and benefits. While being satisfied is essential, it is not enough. Staff must feel energized and be willing to put effort into their work. They must also feel that the work has a purpose and is productive in that their efforts contribute to the overall vision and bottom line of the organization. Vick Hess, an expert in nurse engagement, defines engagement as the emotional and intellectual commitment of an individual to build and sustain business performance. She has simplified this definition into a three-part formula (Figure 7-1). [3]

FIGURE 7-1 THE ENGAGEMENT FORMULA

Satisfied

+

Energized

+

Productive at Work

=

Employee Engagement

One of the most compelling reasons to become a nurse leader coach is the impact that coaching can have on nurse engagement. Your staff wants an authentic relationship with their manager that includes talk about both work *and* life. They want to work somewhere that values their strengths and invests in their ongoing development. Gallup researchers have studied thousands of managers in hundreds of industries worldwide to determine what they do to foster high staff engagement. The best managers all share certain traits: [4]

- They enjoy learning about their team members' strengths.
- They purposefully discover what motivates each person.
- They match talent to task.
- They trust workers to do their best.
- They get out of their workers' way.

Staff engaged in their work have been noted to exhibit passion, commitment and a willingness to invest in themselves to help their organizations succeed. Work engagement has been found to be higher among nurses working for nurse managers who practice authentic leadership, are approachable and are themselves engaged in their work. Workload, level of organizational change, decision latitude and career development opportunities have been found to have an impact on levels of engagement along with the level of job stress. The ability to effectively engage employees is now recognized as an important business differentiator. In healthcare, it has been shown to impact the quality of care, patient satisfaction, and safety.

Engagement Begins with the Leader

Engagement starts with the nurse leader coach. If you are not engaged in your work, it will be impossible to engage staff. Gallup research data indicates that managers account for 70% of the variance in employee engagement, and that US managers are only slightly more engaged in their work than their staff.[5] This is essential data for nurse leaders because your engagement profoundly affects the engagement of your staff.

You need to walk the talk of engagement. Managers who feel overwhelmed sometimes shut down and disengage from their work. That happened to Cathy. Her unit merged with a second unit six months ago. She now manages both units. She has gone being from being a confident leader to feeling like she is drowning. In talking with her mentor, she realized that she had changed nothing about her work patterns although her responsibility had doubled. She had not asked for help and felt herself disengaging from work as a defense mechanism. When this occurs, it is time for the leader to set boundaries and ask themselves what they could stop doing. Like the messages we often hear on airplanes, we need to put our own oxygen masks on first.

Engagement in work requires positive energy and optimism. Author Jon Gordon is well known for his work *The Energy Bus*.[6] He makes a strong point that we all have choices in life whether to be a positive thinker or a negative thinker. Positive thinking starts with the leader.

Using the metaphor of a bus driver, he provides the following ten rules for leaders to fuel their work, their life and their team with positive energy:

Rule 1 – You Are the Driver of Your Bus

Positivity starts with a clear vision for your life, work, and relationships. If you want a good life, rewarding work, and strong relationships, you need to invest your energy to ensure that it happens.

Rule 2 – Desire, Vision, and Focus Move Your Bus in the Right Direction

Gordon believes that you attract what you focus on. If you are negative and think that things won't get better, you will be right.

Rule 3 – Fuel Your Bus with Positive Energy

Staff love positive leaders and become discouraged when leaders are negative. Positive energy is high octane fuel for any team. The more positive you are, the more positive things become.

Rule 4 – Invite People on Your Bus and Share Your Vision for the Future

No leader can work alone. You need your team to help make things work.

Rule 5 – Don't Waste Your Time on People Who Don't Get on the Bus

Too often, leaders spend all their time with their most negative staff trying to get them to be more engaged. Engagement is a choice and not one you can make for anyone else.

Rule 6 – No Energy Vampires Allowed on Your Bus

You build a culture around what you tolerate. Gordon suggests that we should not tolerate negativity. For many staff, it has become a destructive habit. Call it out.

Rule 7 – Enthusiasm Attracts More Passengers and Energizes Them During the Ride

Being around happy and positive people makes everyone else feel happy and positive. Patients can sense when there is positivity on a unit, it changes everything.

Rule 8 – Love Your Passengers

Leaders need to demonstrate that they care deeply about their staff. To love your team, you need to make time for them, listen to them, recognize them, serve them and bring out the very best in them.

Rule 9 – Drive with Purpose

Staff gets inspired when they see the purpose in their work, and have leaders who consistently make connections between what the team does and the outcomes that are achieved.

Rule 10 – Have Fun and Enjoy the Ride

Too many people believe that they will live forever, but no one does. Reflect more, find more moments of joy, take more risks, and leave a legacy in the people that you serve. Using the metaphor of a bus can inspire your leadership and your own energy level.

Measuring Engagement – The Gallup Q12

You may not know the true engagement level of your staff without measuring it. One of the most widely used scales to measure staff engagement is the Gallup Q12. [5] The scale has been in use for more than 15 years and has been subjected to rigorous testing to ensure that it is a valid tool. It measures staff engagement using a 12-element survey with a Likert scale score of 1 to 5. It is rooted in an employee's performance development needs in four areas: basic needs, individual needs, teamwork needs, and personal growth needs. Of the 12 questions on the Gallup Q12, the following six have been found by Gallup to be the most powerful regarding links to employee engagement and multiple other outcomes:

Q1 – I know what is expected of me at work.

Q2 – I have the materials and equipment that I need to do my work.

Q3 – At work, I have the opportunity to do what I do best every day.

Q4 – In the last seven days, I have received recognition or praise for doing good work.

Q5 – My supervisor or someone at work seems to care about me as a person.

Q6 – There is someone at work who encourages my development.

Working with Your Results

Gallup experts recommend that if you want to improve engagement and outcomes that you should focus specific attention on these six items.[5] They use the metaphor of mountain climbing to describe how to approach the journey of improvement. The base of the mountain would include the first two questions in the Gallup Q12 – also described as "Base Camp." Like the bottom of Maslow's Hierarchy of Needs, these are things that employees need to know or have to do their jobs. Gallup research has demonstrated that the highest performing managers are extremely clear about performance goals. They work with each staff member to help them understand how their role contributes to accomplishing those goals.

Once these basic needs are met, managers can focus on the items in Q3–Q6 or what is described as Camp 1. In this camp, managers need to work hard to identify the strengths of each staff member and assign responsibilities to allow their staff to do their best (Q3). The role of recognition and praise for work well done cannot be overemphasized, and it needs to come directly from the manager (Q4). Taking the time to know each employee individually can be challenging, but it is critical if staff are to perceive that they are being cared for and valued for who they are (Q5). Q6 is about a manager who invests in your growth. We know from research with Millennials that coaching and development is a significant retention strategy, so it is a wise investment of a manager's time.

While the other six questions in the Gallup Q12 are an important guide to meeting a staff member's higher-level needs, the best investment is spending time in the areas addressed in Q1–Q6. Gallup research indicates that while Q7–Q12 scores are important when Q1–Q6 scores are low, this suggests level of disengagement that could ultimately result in staff turnover.[5] In the end what matters is that the manager selects the right staff then sets expectations and helps to motivate and develop staff members to higher levels of performance. Questions with low scores provide opportunities for managers to design action plans and strategies to improve engagement. The challenge with employee engagement is that it is not a one and done strategy. Scores can change over time.

Anne, an oncology outpatient clinic manager, discovered this as she reviewed her yearly Q12 scores for the unit. Anne's team had high engagement scores during most of her five-year leadership tenure. This year, the Q12 ratings had plummeted in the areas of meeting staff individual and growth needs. Anne was concerned to see that the score on Q5 (my supervisor or someone at work seems to care about me as a person) had changed from a 4.6 last year to a 3.1 this year. In reflecting on the past year, Anne realized that she had spent a great deal of time off the unit planning a replacement clinic facility. At the same time, she had several new staff members join the team, and had not provided them with the coaching that she usually did as part of the onboarding process. Anne decided that a reboot would be necessary. She began with a staff meeting where she shared the survey results along with her disappointment and desire to improve. She engaged her staff in conversations asking questions such as:

- What makes you feel like a valued member of the team?
- What can I do to let you know that I care about your accomplishments?
- How do you like to be shown that I care and have respect for you?

INVEST IN STRENGTHS

An important strategy to engage staff is to know and encourage staff to use their strengths in their work. Investing in strengths can have a huge payback in the level of staff engagement. Gallup research indicates that seven in ten employees (67%) who strongly agree that their manager focuses on their strengths are engaged in their work. When employees strongly disagree with this statement, the percentage of workers who are engaged in their work plummets to 2%.[7] High engagement translates into higher profitability, better customer satisfaction, and lower turnover. When employees use their strengths, they have been shown to be six times more engaged in their work and 7.8% more productive in their role.

Historically, performance management models have focused on fixing staff weaknesses or deficits. While managing gaps to meet role expectations does matter, part of the joy of being human is the recognition that we are all different and have unique gifts. Everyone has strengths and weakness. When coaching employees, Gallup research has found that the world's greatest managers' report that they don't waste their time focusing on employee weaknesses but instead draw out their talents.[5] This is counter-intuitive to what most managers believe when they have the same expectations in every area for all their staff.

Ideally, organizations would use talent assessments such as the Clifton Strength Finders ® to learn about the unique gifts of their staff.[8] If this is not available, nurse leader coaches can observe their staff to learn about their natural talents and use good coaching questions. Questions to ask to discover talent include:

1. What do you do best in your role?
2. What do you enjoy most about the work you do every day?
3. What do you look forward to doing each day at work?
4. What hobbies do you have?

These questions will give the nurse leader coach insight into the natural talents of staff so they can individualize their approach to enhance the work experience. Janet used this approach with her hospice staff. She learned that Matt, one of her newer team members, had a unique gift to establish trusting relationships with patients and their families quickly. This proved useful in several situations where Janet was able to assign Matt to cases where there was family disagreement about whether the patient should be placed on hospice. With his strength as a relator, he was able to quickly gain the confidence of families who had presented significant challenges to the hospice team.

Engagement as a Joint Responsibility

While nurse leaders play a crucial role in staff engagement, staff also have a personal responsibility to work on their own engagement. Work engagement is a two-way street. Nurse leaders can create environments that engage and empower staff, but they cannot force engagement. Two employees can have very different experiences within the same organization. Engagement ultimately comes from within, and how we view our circumstances. It is essential for the individual to have a clear sense of what makes them engaged or not engaged at work, and what actions they can take to change their situation. Marshall Goldsmith, in his book *Triggers,* observed that survey questions are often asked in a passive voice, such as those in Gallup Q12.[9] This promotes the idea that employee engagement is an organizational responsibility.

The variance sometimes seen in employee engagement may be because some individuals naturally accept their responsibility in the process. Goldsmith promotes the idea that when managers have staff that is not engaged, they should encourage reflection with coaching questions such as:

1. Did I do my best to set clear goals today?
2. Did I do my best to finding meaning in my work today?
3. Did I do my best to happy today?
4. Did I do my best to build positive relationships today?
5. Did I do my best to be fully engaged today?

These questions encourage the idea of action learning as part of the engagement process by emphasizing a need for ongoing growth and reflection. All of us have a strong need to be respected, recognized for our talents, feel a sense of belonging and do work that we think is essential. Only an individual staff member can truly know whether they are happy at work and if not, does something need to change. Nurse leaders can create an environment for staff happiness and engagement, but may find that some staff is still unhappy. That is not the nurse leader's responsibility, and it never can be.

Remember

✓ The ability to effectively engage staff is an important business differentiator.

✓ One of the most compelling reasons to become a nurse leader coach is the impact that coaching can have on nurse engagement.

✓ Nurse leaders account for 70% of the variance in staff engagement. Engagement starts with an engaged leader.

✓ Nurse leaders can create environments that engage and empower staff, but they cannot force engagement.

CHAPTER 8

Master Good Communication

One of the most powerful skills that a leader coach can have is excellent communication. We see it in sports teams. When you watch great coaches in action, they seem to know just what to say to their star players at the right time to motivate them. They recognize the importance of individualizing their communication to the needs of each player. When providing this continuous feedback, they build the foundation and trust to have tough conversations under pressure.

New nurse leaders are often surprised about how challenging communication is in today's environment. Research from the Center for Creative Leadership has also found that communication is one of the skills that new leaders struggle with more often than others. [10] As a leader, you are always communicating either verbally or nonverbally. The frontline nurse leader role has been compared to an air traffic controller because you are at the center of communication flow on your unit. You are seen as a pivotal point person, or 'go to' person. You must master the art of assertive and persuasive communication, as well as develop negotiation and listening skills. Your success in communication efforts as a leader coach is reflected in staff, patient, and physician satisfaction scores. Poor communication is the root cause of most sentinel events and medical errors. It is always better to err on the side of too much versus too little communication.

COMMUNICATION STARTS WITH LISTENING

Nurse leaders often build their early career success by having all the answers. This changes when you move into a leadership role. You will not have all the answers and should move to deeper listening to the viewpoints of others. As a nurse leader coach, it can be difficult to know what employees think unless you take the time to sit down and listen to them. Tanya learned this lesson in her first year of leadership. When she started in her role, staff would come into her office with a problem. She would immediately jump into action without really listening to the whole conversation. However, in most situations, her staff just wanted to vent about a situation and did not expect her to act or even give them advice. They wanted to be heard. So, she learned to shift what she does in these conversations. She had to tame the advice monster in her and ask *is this a problem that you would like my help with or do you just want to tell me about it and vent.* She was moving from being "a manager in charge of all issues" to a leader coach. She could not do it without becoming a better listener.

Michael Bungay Stanier, an expert leadership coach, recommends that to tame the advice monster in you—ask better questions and make them open-ended even when every fiber in your body is dying to solve the problem.[11] This involves a change in behavior especially when you have the advice monster habit. The right questions will open the door to discovery and a more open dialogue with others. To become a better listener, consider implementing these five strategies:

1. **Be fully present** – Leaders need to be fully present when engaged in a conversation to understand what is being said. This means no multitasking. Don't read email or text message and ignore phone calls unless urgent. It also means not focusing on your response to what is being said.

2. **Ask open-ended clarifying questions** – Michael Bungay Stanier has some great suggestions for open-ended questions in conversations with staff. *What's on Your Mind? (then be silent and listen) And What Else? (avoid being an advice monster) What is the real challenge here for you? What do you want? How can I help?*[11]

3. **Avoid being an advice monster** – Leaders often see themselves as experts and feel compelled to be the expert and offer a solution to a problem right away. The problem is that we can jump to conclusions and suggest what should be done before the other person has fully explained his or her perspective?

4. **Embrace silence** – Aim to talk no more than 20% of the time in a conversation. Don't feel obligated to respond to every comment. If there is a lull in the conversation – be OK with it. Sometimes the most profound thoughts will follow.

5. **Enter every conversation with the assumption that you will learn something** – See conversations as a way to gain insight and knowledge that you don't already have rather than an imposition on your time. If you believe that there is something to be learned, it will be a self-fulfilling prophecy.

Thoughtful questions will open the door to discovery and a more open dialogue with others. Thoughtful open-ended questions help move the relationship from the traditional manager who tells staff what to do to a leader coach. Although it may seem that providing our staff with answers to their problems is the most efficient way to get things done, it does not foster growth. A coaching approach forces you to make the conversation less about you and more about the staff member. Judith Ross suggests that the most useful questions create value. [12] The following are some great examples:

1. **To create clarity** – Can you explain more about this situation? What do you think the issue is here?
2. **To help staff think analytically and more critically** – What are the consequences if you take this action? If our organization does not take action to decrease our financial costs, what will happen when reimbursements decline?
3. **To inspire reflection** – Why do you think you were successful in that situation? What is different about today's healthcare environment that when you initially began your career?
4. **To encourage breakthrough thinking** – Is there another way that we could do this? If you were redesigning care today with a blank slate, what type of delivery system would you develop?
5. **To challenge assumptions** – What would happen if we fail to take action given what is happening with health reform? Do you think that this type of care needs to be delivered in a hospital setting?
6. **To create ownership of solutions** – Based on your nursing experience, what do you suggest that we do here? What changes would be in the best interest of your patients?

Start with Why

Effective communication should be open, clear and timely. Much of the communication in healthcare today involves changes in policies, procedures, and practices. How we deliver messages especially if we are asking staff to change will impact the effectiveness of the communication. The conventional pathway used by leaders to communicate change is to start with what will change, and then explain how it will change. Simon Sinek, a leadership and communications expert, cautions that this is the wrong approach especially with the Millennial workforce who want transparency in communication about change. To achieve remarkable results, Sinek explains that this order needs to be changed and leaders need to begin by explaining why there is a need for change before they talk about what will change and how it will change. (Figure 8-1) [13]

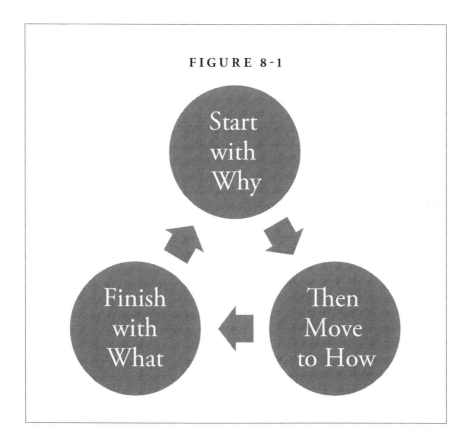

FIGURE 8-1

Start with Why

Then Move to How

Finish with What

Start with the Why

The **why** of your communication should include the sense of urgency behind the change and potential impact to the organization without the change. A documentation policy may need to be revised because of changes in reimbursement. A health system may need to close a patient unit because of declining patient volumes. A nurse manager may need to alter an already posted staffing schedule because of significant changes in patient acuity.

Move to the How

In the current healthcare environment, many organizations have financial challenges, and leaders are being asked to implement new strategies to meet the demands of changes coming with health reform. This may result in changes in **how** you do what you do. Your how today is likely to involve designing strategies to provide the right patient the right care at the right time in the right place and at the right price.

Finish with the What

The **what** or goal should come last not first. Nursing staff needs the context of the why and how before they hear the procedural and policy changes that impact their practice. What is it that you want them to do differently in their work.

Then Help Them Remember

There is so much communication in most organizations that messages can be easily lost. You need to build a strategy to help staff to easily remember what has been communicated especially vital changes. Some managers use physical message boards or send group texts. Others place key communication in staff restrooms and lockers. One creative manager bakes cupcakes, and places them on index cards with information about upcoming changes on the unit.

Evidence-Based Communication Tools

Communication in healthcare environments can be challenging. There are so many different team members that work with patients. Clarity in communication is critical. Fortunately, there are useful tools available to help communicate more effectively, and even more important to make sure the communication is understood. Strategies and Tools to Enhance Performance and Patient Safety (TeamSTEPPS) is an evidence-based communication model that has been developed for use in clinical practice with funding from the Agency for Healthcare Research and Quality. Although these tools were developed for the use of clinicians to communicate with one another, they are also excellent tools for a leader to coach staff. Tools in the model include the Two-Challenge Rule, Call-Outs, and Check-Backs. [14]

The Two-Challenge Rule – requires the communicator to voice their concern at least twice to receive acknowledgment by the receiver. This rule may be invoked when a member of the healthcare team suggests or performs an intervention that deviates from the standard of care. The nurse leader would assertively voice their concern at least two times, and if the team member who is being challenged does not acknowledge this concern, the leader would then take a stronger action or utilize the hospital chain of command as needed.

Call-Outs – are a strategy that the leaders can use to inform all team members of crucial information during emergencies to assist team members in anticipating what comes next. For instance, during a stroke alert, the results of the patient's NIH scale and the need to transport the patient as rapidly as possible for a CT scan may be communicated out loud to the rest of the team.

Check-Back's – require the sender of the communication to verify the information that is being received by the other team member, or to use closed-loop communication. For example, the nurse leader is responsible for verifying that changes in practice are being implemented and performed according to policy.

Words have Power in Leadership

Nurse leaders speak in an amplified voice. Staff pay close attention to the messages that are sent by leaders and requests that are made. Casual comments are easily misinterpreted. Ralph learned this the hard way. He returned from a senior leadership meeting held to discuss patient throughput in the emergency department where he was the manager.

His charge nurse asked him how things went and he told her that it had not gone well. "*They don't get what we do here at all—it is very frustrating.*" He later heard his words echoed in a staff conversation and immediately regretted shifting the blame to the administrative staff. Words used by leaders can either signal a high degree of optimism, inclusiveness and teamwork or they can make a leader appear mistrustful and self-centered.

If a leader is definitive in their language advising staff with words such as "your jobs are secure" or "you will definitely be able to do this" then you need to be prepared to deliver on these promises. Words can build up the self-esteem of followers or they can cause pain, anger, frustration and emotional withdrawal. Successful leaders understand the power of words and choose words to do the following:

1. Create a Culture of Inclusiveness

The pronouns used by leaders can help build a culture of inclusiveness. Excessive use of the word *they* on a team is a sign of problems with harmony and teamwork. It also characterizes environments where there is blame game going on. Instead of *"they,"* leaders need to shift the language to the pronoun *"we."* It is one of the most important words in leadership language. It is inclusive, builds a team culture and helps to break down silos in organizations. Never describe anyone as "just a staff nurse."

2. Encourage Others

Words that are affirming help to make people feel good. Encouraging words help to get others through difficult times. Leaders who excessively use the word *"I"* instead of *"we"* may be taking more credit than they deserve in situations. Leaders also need to be careful about their use of the possessive pronoun *my* to describe *"my unit"* or *"my team."* This can imply a level of ownership that others may resent.

3. Build Relationships

Building relationships with others is a crucial leadership skill. Words that recognize the contributions and strengths of others help to create positive relationships. Every leader has probably had the experience of using just the right words in a relationship to help it grow or using the wrong choice of words that made the situation worse. Some choices of words that can be damaging when working with a staff member are: *"What you NEED to do…", "What you SHOULD do…", "What you MUST do" or "If I were you…. I would"*. These words can completely shut down a conversation.

Learning to choose your words wisely will help you to grow into the type of nurse leader your staff will not want to leave.

Communicating with Staff

Most of us have a preferred method of how we like others to communicate with us. This could be text messages, emails or a phone call. These preferences should be shared with the staff. You should also talk with team members about the timeframe that you will be back in touch with them. Many organizations require staff to have email accounts, and ask their leaders to communicate using email because it establishes a record of conversations. If this is true in your organization, then you are expected to read and respond to your email.

When nurse leaders don't respond to their email or phone messages, it is frustrating for staff and colleagues. It conveys a message that this is not a priority for the leader and does not promote a positive work environment. It can also impact how you are perceived as a leader in a very negative way. Sometimes, leaders don't respond to requests because they don't want to answer negatively but, in many respects, no answer is far worse than a negative response. It exacerbates conflict. Leadership expert, Margaret Hefferman, has noted that how responsive you are to email in today's environment often defines your leadership. She also notes that the following are important to consider: [15]

1. Your response time to email or phone message is a non-verbal cue about your leadership behavior. Research shows that the longer you take to respond, the more negatively you are viewed as a leader.
2. Replying to email or other messages is simple politeness; ignoring them suggests that you don't care about the issue or the person who wrote to you. It's virtually impossible to have good working relationships if your silence contains, or even hints at contempt.
3. How you deal with requests or messages says something fundamental about how reliable you are. And that translates into trust.

4. Reputations are built as an outcome of many small actions. It's easy to think that small actions don't matter and, individually, they might not. However, cumulatively your daily behavior is what people notice and like or dislike, trust or distrust.

5. You can actually build an excellent reputation and even fame by just being responsive to requests from others.

6. Thinking that no response is the new no is, in fact, passive aggressive and rude. Most people can handle rejection far better than not knowing.

Nurse leaders should make responsiveness to messages and requests a priority. Recognize that response time says volumes about your character. If you are busy, just acknowledge the email and let them know you will get back to them. If you miss an email, apologize and acknowledge it. Improving your email and phone etiquette will enhance your leadership reputation in ways that you might not anticipate.

COMMUNICATING ON EMAIL

Few nurse leaders can't tell you a story about an email that they wished they had not sent. A poorly written email, an email sent in anger or even the inclusion of a cute cartoon that is misinterpreted can have unintended negative consequences. Jake recognized this problem when one of his charge nurses sent a very negative email to the director of the laboratory. It was full of accusations and seemed way out of proportion to the incident that provoked it. As an outcome of the email, Jake had to do significant damage control with the laboratory and performance coaching with the charge nurse. Email etiquette is vital in any nursing leadership role. Before you send that email, ask yourself the following questions:

1. **WHAT AM I TRYING TO ACHIEVE IN SENDING THIS EMAIL?**
   Emails are time-consuming to read. Before you send an email, ask yourself what you are trying to achieve and formulate a short but to the point message. Emails containing nonwork-related stories or jokes are often annoying to recipients and waste time.

2. **IS AN EMAIL THE RIGHT FORM OF COMMUNICATION FOR THIS MESSAGE?**
   It is easy to misinterpret information that is communicated in email messages. Misunderstandings that could quickly be cleared up in a face to face conversation or by phone can quickly escalate in email exchanges. Email can be a great way to commend someone but is rarely the right way to address performance issues. If you need to discuss a controversial subject, an email may not be the best way to do this. You can unintentionally create a firestorm of conflict.

3. **AM I ANGRY AS I WRITE THIS?**
   Emails that are written in the heat of anger are rarely effective nor is capitalizing words for emphasis. Accusatory or nasty emails can be career limiting so wait 24 hours before you send an email if you are angry.

4. **IS THIS EMAIL BEING SENT ONLY TO PEOPLE WHO NEED THIS INFORMATION?**
   The volume of email is escalating throughout all work environments. Recipients understandably get inpatient with unnecessary emails. Use the cc field sparingly and only include people on the message who have a need to know. Don't send the message as a high priority unless it is critical communication.

5. **Does the email have a subject that will get the attention of the reader?**

   A strong subject line will grab the attention of the reader and make it more likely that your email will be read. Emails with a blank subject line sometimes are inadvertently deleted by busy recipients who scan their incoming mail.

6. **Is my message brief and to the point?**

   Email messages that are too long, poorly-written or ineffective in conveying their purpose can cause confusion, unnecessary back-and-forth, loss of time and productivity, and frustration. A good email should get the response and the result you desire while presenting yourself in the best possible way. Write your email messages in two or three paragraphs. Make sure your intent is clear and conveys a purpose. Do you need action from the recipient or are you giving information? Emails should contain both a personalized greeting and your signature line.

7. **Have I checked the email for grammar and spelling?**

   Carefully check your emails for grammar and spelling. The content of messages that are full of errors can be easily lost as the recipient focuses on grammar and spelling errors. Always read the email you typed before you send it. Make sure the font is large enough to read and avoid colored backgrounds on your messages.

8. **Would I feel good about this email if it was presented in court as evidence in a case?**

   Email messages that you write are a permanent written record of your communication. Once you send the email, you can no longer control who sees the message. Work emails can and are used in court cases against employers. If a staff member has a performance issue, leaders need to be very careful about what they write in their emails. Likewise, emails about problems with patient safety and quality should also be avoided.

Leadership Visibility

Nurse leader coaches who want to establish strong communication with staff need to be visible. It is impossible to successfully lead from behind your desk. You need to be intentional in planning time to talk with staff. This is a challenge for nurse managers today who struggle with large spans of control and increased administrative responsibilities. Yet, no one wants to be led by someone who rarely if ever comes out of his or her office. Visibility in leadership matters. The following are three strategies that you can use to improve your leadership visibility:

1. **Purposeful Leadership Rounding**
   Purposeful nurse leader rounding on patients is quickly becoming a best practice in hospitals throughout the United States. When it is done well, it can have a positive direct impact on both patients and staff. It has been shown to improve both patient and staff satisfaction. It is an organized way for nurse leaders to be visible in their areas of responsibility which can lead to an openness with staff that will build trust and facilitates communication. Quick coaching conversations can occur during rounding. As a leader, you learn what is working well in your unit and department, and where there may be a need for improvement. It provides an excellent opportunity to scan the environment for equipment and supply issues that concern staff. Nurses sometimes have the impression that when times get tough – their leaders withdraw. That is why consistency in rounding is so important and should be a regular part of every leader's schedule.

2. NURSE MANAGER FIVE MINUTE HUDDLES

There is so much changing in today's environment that nursing staff can become quite anxious if a nurse manager isolates him/herself in their office. Brief daily huddles can be a great way to update the team on changes. How leaders use language to frame people, situations, and events has significant consequences for the way individuals make sense of the world and their actions. Not all nurse leaders think about this when they communicate, but it is crucial. The response of leaders to change or turbulence in their environment has a powerful effect on their staff. Leaders who remain calm, truthful and optimistic in their communications help to prevent the spread of misinformation and reduce staff anxiety. The words and non-verbal behaviors of leaders can be very powerful in a positive or a negative way.

3. OPEN YOUR OFFICE DOOR AND BE APPROACHABLE

Leaving your office door open at least some of the time sounds like an obvious strategy but one that is often not used. Some nurse managers may worry that they will experience constant interruptions if they leave the door open. However if you make it a practice to leave the door open when you are available, most staff will be respectful of your time. Having your office door open is not enough; you must also appear approachable to staff, so they are comfortable walking in and having a conversation. No matter how challenged you are timewise; you cannot lead from behind the desk. Make time to be visible, to be seen and to listen.

BECOME A STORY TELLER

Nursing leadership is about influence and persuasion. Storytelling is a useful tool to persuade others. Nurse leaders use storytelling every day whether we consciously think about it or not. A story can be used in coaching to simulate the experience. Using stories can trump facts because they humanize the problem. As a nurse leader, you may coach staff in fall prevention and try to summon a sense of urgency for initiatives such as patient rounding. You may find that it is much more powerful to take one patient situation where there was a bad outcome from a fall. You can tell the story of how the fall impacted that patient's life. At the conclusion of the story present, the information about the number of falls is occurring on the unit each month.

As leaders, it is important to give staff encouragement during difficult times. Sandra saw this in her leader coaching. One of her new graduate staff nurses incorrectly transcribed a verbal order that resulted in a medication error. She was devastated by the mistake. Sandra shared her own experience with a similar error, and talked about what she had learned from it. When leaders share vulnerability, they gain respect. This young nurse was amazed that her manager who seemed so competent had once made a similar mistake.

Effective coaching stories have the following five key elements:

1. They are context specific and fit the topic that is being discussed.
2. They consider the position of the staff member and their career stage.
3. They are told by respected role models.
4. They have drama and draw the listener's attention.
5. They have high learning value and are a call to change behavior.

Through the effective use of story, nurse leaders can both build strong cultures and connect with staff at a personal level.

REMEMBER

✓ As a leader, you are always communicating either verbally or nonverbally.

✓ To tame the advice monster in you – ask better questions and make them open-ended even when every fiber in your body is dying to solve the problem.

✓ Your response time to messages and requests says volumes about your leadership.

✓ It is impossible to effectively lead from behind your desk if you are not intentional in planning time to leave your office and talk with staff.

CHAPTER 9

NAVIGATE CONFLICT

Work teams today are composed of staff from different generations with divergent values, attitudes, and beliefs. These differences can and do lead to conflict. The level of conflict also increases when the pace of change accelerates, so it is not surprising that we do see more of it in today's turbulent healthcare environment. While some conflict is inevitable, elevating the conflict to the level of drama is a choice and one that should not occur in work environments. What is different in healthcare is that when conflict is not managed well, the outcomes of unresolved problems can become a patient safety issue.

While conflict is central to all interactions because of the diversity of human experience, it can be time-consuming to work through issues. Nurse leaders report that they spend a great deal of time coaching staff through conflict situations. The good news is that while conflict situations were once thought of as a bad thing, we now realize that they can help us to grow and reach common ground more quickly if we manage them well. It can serve as a positive driving force for change and improvement. When staff members are coached to manage conflict effectively, they can move past differences and avoid making the conflict destructive. To effectively coach staff in conflict situations, it is essential to recognize that different people have different conflict management styles and may need to learn how to debate issues constructively.

Conflict Management Styles

Not everyone manages conflict in the same way. Although many of us can flex our style when needed, we usually have a preferred method of handling conflict which is important to identify. According to the widely used Thomas Kilmann Conflict Resolution Model, there are five primary modes of managing conflict: *avoiding, accommodating, competing, collaboration and compromising.*[17]

- **Competing** is defined as an assertive and uncooperative approach to conflict where the individual pursues his or her own concerns at the other person's expense. This is a power-oriented mode in which you use whatever power seems appropriate to win your position—your ability to argue, your rank, or economic sanctions. Competing means "standing up for your rights," defending a position that you believe is correct, or merely trying to win.
- **Accommodating** is defined as an unassertive and cooperative approach to managing conflict. It is the complete opposite of competing. When accommodating, the individual neglects his or her concerns to satisfy the interests of the other person; there is an element of self-sacrifice in this mode. Accommodating might take the form of selfless generosity, obeying another person's order when you would prefer not to, or yielding to another's point of view.

- **Avoiding** is an unassertive and uncooperative response to conflict where the person neither pursues his or her concerns nor those of the other individual. Thus, he or she does not deal with the conflict. Avoiding might take the form of diplomatically sidestepping an issue, postponing an issue until a better time, or simply withdrawing from a threatening situation. In my own leadership work, I have found that many nurses use this approach when in stressful conflict situations.
- **Collaborating** is both an assertive and cooperative response to conflict, and is the complete opposite of avoiding. Collaborating involves an attempt to work with others to find a solution that fully satisfies their concerns. It means digging into an issue to pinpoint the underlying needs and wants of the two individuals. Collaborating with two persons might take the form of exploring a disagreement to learn from each other's insights or trying to find a creative solution to an interpersonal problem.
- **Compromising** is a moderate response in both assertiveness and cooperativeness. The objective is to find some expedient, mutually acceptable solution that partially satisfies both parties. It falls between competing and accommodating. Compromising gives up more than competing but less than accommodating. Likewise, it addresses an issue more directly than avoiding but does not explore it in as much depth as collaborating. In some situations, compromising might mean splitting the difference between the two positions, exchanging concessions, or seeking a quick middle-ground solution.

ASKING THE RIGHT QUESTIONS

We can develop the capability of using all five modes of conflict-resolution. The key is to choose the right approach for the right situation to be effective. Jennifer, the manager of a large primary care clinic, was surprised to learn when she took the Thomas-Kilmann assessment that her preferred mode of managing conflict was to compete. Upon reflection, she had to acknowledge that this was how she approached conflict. Jennifer was by nature a competitive person who enjoyed winning arguments. Her director had talked with her about her combative style when she disagreed with others. She was fighting every battle in the same way, and needed to flex her conflict management approaches to the situation. Ultimately if she failed to manage conflict differently, Jennifer realized it could derail her leadership. She needed to be more thoughtful in conflict situations and ask better questions to gain clarity before she took the next step. Some examples of questions she could have asked include the following:

WHAT ARE THE BACKGROUND ISSUES DRIVING THE CONFLICT?

Experts contend that there are always antecedents to any conflict situation. Before a leader intervenes in a conflict, they need to assess how and why it is happening now. The antecedent conditions are what started the conflict. An example of this is when a charge nurse changes the assignment of staff nurse during the shift because of unexpected admissions and discharges. This can then lead to conflict if the staff nurse disagrees with the assignment change. Assessing the administrative decisions or personal relationship issues that led to a conflict could be essential to consider in conflict resolution.

IS THE CONFLICT ESCALATING OR WILL IT EVENTUALLY RESOLVE ITSELF?

Not every conflict needs to be managed, yet some do escalate very quickly without intervention. How you resolve a dispute involving a patient's family knowing the patient will be discharged tomorrow will be different from conflict between two team members who need to work together. While avoidance might be the right approach if the patient will soon be discharged, it might not be for staff working on the same team, and who are in conflict with one another.

When, where and how should I take appropriate action?

In some conflict situations, it will be appropriate to coach staff to resolve their own conflict. In more serious or escalating situations, the nurse leader coach will need to become personally involved. To be effective especially in escalating situations, how the conflict is managed needs to be intentional and specific steps need to be followed.

Steps in Mediating a Conflict

The following steps in the conflict resolution process can be used to help staff discuss and mediate the conflict that involves differences:

1. **Bring the individuals in conflict together to address the problem.**

   As a first step, you need to bring individuals together who are in conflict with one another. They may resist this and want to tell their stories to you in private but if you allow this you risk polarizing their positions. You need to make sure that all parties concerned are participating together in the discussion. These conversations should not be a one-sided monologue.

2. **Agree to ground rules for discussion that are acceptable to all parties.**

   As the mediator of the conflict, it will be helpful to establish some ground rules regarding the discussion. These ground rules could include no interrupting, no personal attacks and no discussion of issues unrelated to this specific conflict.

3. **LET EACH PERSON CLARIFY HIS OR HER PERSPECTIVE AND OPINION ON THE ISSUE.**

Allow each person to tell their story from their perspective. Applying a time limit to the discussion may be helpful. Doing so helps each person speak about the issues that matter and reduces the conversational clutter that has little bearing on the conflict.

4. **HIGHLIGHT SOME COMMON GROUND THAT ALL INVOLVED IN THE CONFLICT CAN AGREE ON.**

Common ground in conflict is significant because it can serve a reference point to help bring the discussion back on track. As an example, most staff can agree that they are there to provide the best possible care to patients. When conflict escalates, you can bring the individuals back to this point of common ground.

5. **DEVELOP INTERVENTIONS COLLABORATIVELY AND AGREE TO DISAGREE ON POINTS OF CONTENTION.**

Holding desperately to a dogmatic grudge isn't likely to yield many benefits in workplace conflict. Presenting a conflict as a black-or-white, right-or-wrong situation heightens tension. Work to help the individuals develop interventions collaboratively. Identify the points of major contention; it may be necessary to agree to disagree.

6. **KEEP THE LINES OF COMMUNICATION OPEN AND RESPECT DIFFERENCES IN ATTITUDES, VALUES, AND BEHAVIORS.**

The goal in most conflicts will be to open the lines of communication and re-establish working relationships. Try not to take someone's conflicting opinion as a negative assessment of you as a person or as a co-worker. It can help to acknowledge the differences in attitudes, values, and beliefs openly.

Your overall objective in the mediation of conflict should be able to help team members work more effectively together to meet the needs of patients. Keep in mind that the conflict never just impacts the people involved. Team members and employees with whom the conflicting employees interact are affected by the stress. Conflict and mediation always contain opportunities for staff growth. Some interesting post-conflict coaching questions could include:

- How did you grow from this situation?
- What did your reactions in this situation reveal about you as a professional?
- What did you learn from this situation that could prevent it from happening again?

Carefronting to Manage Conflict

A different approach to manage conflict is to think of it as *carefronting*. The term *carefronting was* coined by David Augsburger, a professor of pastoral care, more than three decades ago. [18] Dr. Augsburger believes that conflict is to be expected. It is the way that it is managed that impacts the relationships. In carefronting, personal needs are integrated with the wants and needs of others. The overall goal is to attain and maintain effective, productive working relationships. Carefronting is a method of communication that entails caring enough about one's self, one's goals, and others to confront courageously in a self-asserting, responsible manner. [19] The following are some fundamental principles:

1. Seek the Truth

When there is a genuine interest in seeking the truth, leaders demonstrate the willingness and ability to listen to others with empathy, and a desire to understand their viewpoint. The goal is to be accurate in what is heard but also being honest with one's feelings and attitudes. It is demonstrating that you care about the relationship.

2. Own your Anger

Anger is often a natural part of the conflict. When anger is acknowledged in a constructive way, it can be a positive, self-affirming emotion. If one feels ignored or rejected, the typical response is anger. Letting the other person know that you are a person of worth and demand respect is essential.

3. Invite Change

Carefronting invites changes but does not demand it. When leaders invite change, they should focus on the behavior and not the person. They should make observations and not draw conclusions. They should present descriptions, not judgments. They should offer ideas and alternatives, not only advice and answers. Change should be invited by carefronting in a caring manner, one that is clear but gentle and constructive.

4. Demonstrate Trust

Trust underlies, connects and integrates human emotions. Trust is essential in work relationships. Leaders have to confront situations openly, frankly and responsibly with the viewpoint that the other person will assume his/her responsibility to be equally honest and frank.

5. Stop the Blame

Assigning blame in a conflict inevitably evokes resistance and resentment. Carefronting ends the blame game. Leader coaches can then ask the following questions:

- *What is the respectful thing to do now?*
- *Where do we go from here?*

- *When do we start to discuss the conflict—If not now, when?*
- *Who will end the blame and help work toward the professional practice environment we all deserve?*

6. GET UNSTUCK

Getting unstuck means owning the responsibility for one's role in the conflict. It also involves refusing to waste any additional time in assigning blame.

7. MAKE PEACE

Nurse leaders who are peacemakers are caring people who take the risk to be present in conflict no matter how difficult. They value others and understand their values. They also understand that there are multiple viewpoints in every conflict that need to be appreciated.

The use of carefronting is especially important in health care settings where team synergy and interdependence are required for high quality and safe patient care. Relationships on health care teams live within the contexts of conversations that team members have, or don't have with one another.

WHEN THE CONFLICT IS WITH YOUR BOSS

Managing conflict well is a challenge for most nurse leaders under the best of circumstances. When the conflict is with your boss, it can be difficult and stressful. This was the challenge that Becky faced with her new director of critical care. Her former director had hired her. They had a comfortable relationship and rarely disagreed about how Becky managed situations in the cardiac care unit. However, things had now changed. Becky found herself frequently at odds with her new director who seemed to lack trust in her leadership.

Unless managed well, interpersonal conflict with one's boss and upper management is often a primary issue leading to leadership career derailment. The type of conflict that Becky is facing does not necessarily have to result in resignation, but it will take intentional work to make the relationship better. Sharpe and Johnson in their work *Managing Conflict with your Boss,* describe the following examples of situations that can lead to conflict with one's supervisor: [20]

1. **THERE IS A LACK OF ROLE CLARITY AND ALIGNMENT IN YOUR ROLE.**

   A lack of role clarity may be a source of conflict if your supervisor has expectations that you may feel are not within the scope of your role. This can happen when you are in a position with a matrixed reporting structure to more than one supervisor.

2. **YOU AND YOUR BOSS ARE AT DIFFERENT VANTAGE POINTS.**

   When you and your boss have different viewpoints about what should be the priority in your role, this can lead to conflict. You may be a leader who values close relationships with front-line staff, and your boss wants you to focus more attention on the business strategy or performance metrics.

3. **YOU LACK CONFIDENCE IN YOUR BOSS'S ABILITY.**

   This scenario can happen in situations where nurse leaders serve in interim positions, and then are not selected for the role. They may feel skeptical about the ability of the candidate who was chosen.

4. **YOUR BOSS LACKS CONFIDENCE IN YOU.**

   Sometimes a few missteps early in a relationship can lead to a lack of confidence by your supervisor. You may then find yourself being questioned on every decision.

5. There is a mismatch of values or style.

Leaders tend to be most comfortable with team members that have their same vision, values, and style. If you are different in temperament or style, this can lead to conflict.

Assess Your Role in the Conflict

Before any discussion with your boss about the conflict, it is essential to assess what your role is in the deterioration of the relationship. Ask yourself what your response has been to the conflict. Do you try to keep the lines of communication open and keep your boss informed of your activities? Have you been deeply reflective or are you openly discussing the conflict with others? Are you delivering on the promises that you make? Have you tried to be supportive in meetings? Did you engage in any political maneuvering to take your issues to a higher level? Have you sent any toxic emails? What are your expectations of your supervisor and are they unrealistic? Ask peers close to you who have observed you in interactions with your boss what you could do differently.

Resolving the Conflict

Once you have developed a personal awareness of your role in the conflict, you are now ready to move to the conflict resolution stage. Conflict is best resolved in a face to face setting where both parties feel comfortable. It is often the case that conflict occurs when the lines of communication break down so reopening them is crucial. When discussing the conflict, Sharpe and Johnson recommend that you craft a message to clarify your viewpoints and a desire to build a better relationship.[20] It is also essential that you attempt to understand your supervisor's perspective on the situation. Look for common ground and brainstorm solutions.

Then don't leave without an action plan and a follow-up meeting to discuss progress.

Developing your conflict management skills is like building a muscle. The more you do it, the more effective you will be. As challenging as the conflict is, unresolved conflict can come at a very high cost. Unresolved disputes often lead to a loss of productivity as those involved draw others into their drama. It can lead to the turnover of valuable employees. The competition that can be an outcome of conflict can have a negative impact on team relationships. Those involved in conflict often pay a heavy price in term of their health leading to things like depression, anxiety, and loss of sleep. The biggest losers in unresolved conflict are often patients because conflict leads to communication issues that directly impact the quality of patient care.

REMEMBER:

✓ Where conflict was once thought of as a bad thing, we now realize that it can help us to grow and reach common ground more quickly if we manage it well.
✓ Not everyone manages conflict in the same way.
✓ Carefronting is a different way to view the conflict.
✓ As challenging as the conflict is, unresolved conflict can come at a very high cost.

CHAPTER 10

GIVE CONSTRUCTIVE PERFORMANCE FEEDBACK

There are three different coaching conversations that nurse leaders have with staff. The first involves professional growth where the focus is on helping staff to grow in their professional role. The second context for coaching is nurse career development. This relates to goals that nurses have pertaining to their career progression. The third coaching conversation is directly related to performance management. The goal here is to explore whether and how the staff member is meeting their performance expectations and identifying areas for growth.

Historically, performance conversations were held once a year during the annual evaluation. Ideas about performance management have changed as younger generations in the workforce seek more feedback about how they are doing. Wise managers recognize that frequent performance coaching conversations build the skill sets of staff and increase engagement.

Renee, a surgical manager, has found that short on the spot coaching conversations work well with the nurses on her critical care unit, many of whom are new graduates. It has also proven to be invaluable in building the leadership skills of her staff. Nancy, one of her newer charge nurses, recently asked her for specific feedback about how she is doing in her leadership of the unit. Renee uses a three-part performance feedback framework. The first part is what Renee should *stop doing* in her charge nurse role. This would include one or more factors that get in the way of Renee's effectiveness as a charge nurse. The second part of the discussion is about what is going well, and she should *keep doing*. The last part of the conversation are ideas about behaviors that could make Renee more effective and she should *start doing*. A sample coaching conversation that Renee might use is outlined below:

Stop Doing – I would recommend that to increase teamwork and improve satisfaction on the night shift, you should stop complaining about how much work you have to do.

Keep Doing – Your organizational skills are phenomenal. Continue to track your admissions, transfers, and discharges and make the staffing adjustments needed.

Start Doing – To improve communication on the night shift, I would recommend that you conduct a team huddle at both the beginning and end of the shift.

Constructive coaching feedback if applied well can lead to significant improvements in our performance, but we have to be intentional in how it is given. Some key rules include:

1. **Keep it positive** – performance feedback should consist of what is going well in addition to any needed areas for improvement.

2. **Keep it inclusive** – performance feedback should include the thoughts and ideas of the staff member concerning the issues discussed.

3. **Keep it private** – performance feedback if negative should be given in a secluded area where others can't hear what is being said.

4. **Keep it factual** – performance feedback should be based on observation and fact, not on opinions and gossip.

5. **Keep it specific** – performance feedback should address no more than one to two specific areas of improvement.

6. **Keep it time focused** – performance feedback should include a time when a follow-up conversation will take place.

Performance feedback is essential especially for new graduates who often have difficulty gauging how well they are doing in their role. Kelsey, a medical-surgical manager, encountered this issue on her unit which is home to many new graduates each year. Her seasoned charge nurses frequently complain that the new graduates have poor critical thinking skills yet it is clear to Kelsey that they have received little coaching to become more competent.

Good coaching is critical to the development of strong clinical reasoning. New nurses need to be provided with learning opportunities where a coach helps them through guided discussion and reflection to connect their thinking and action. Some good questions that Kelsey's charge nurses could ask to promote critical thinking skills include the following:

- What is the first thing that you plan to do after receiving a report on your patients?
- What tasks can wait until later?
- What is confusing to you?
- How long can you wait to intervene?
- What are your major concerns with the care of this patient today?

- How will you evaluate the appropriateness of that intervention?
- What could go wrong here?
- What evidence are you using to support your assessment?
- What did you learn from this experience?

Hope and encouragement about the progress that they are making is critical feedback for nurses, especially when it comes from their nurse leaders. [21]

MANAGING PERFORMANCE PROBLEMS

It is easy to be a great nurse leader coach when things are going well, and everyone is performing at his or her highest capability. The real test for a leader is how poor performance is managed. The whole team watches this. When you see poor work, you must address it in a timely way. It should be done privately and positively. You need to show you care, ask good questions, offer practical advice and initiate an action plan. This may take repetition but it needs to be addressed every time, and if there is no change, there need to be ramifications. Good coaches never make this personal but rather ensure it is a professional expectation.

Confronting employees with negative feedback can be uncomfortable, especially for first-time managers. This happened to Ray. Ray is the new director of his emergency department. During his first staff meeting, Sara an experienced nurse was very disrespectful to him. She rolled her eyes at him and lashed out when he introduced a new change to unit policy. It was a painful public moment for Ray. He exercised a great deal of emotional restraint and told Sara that they would discuss her concerns after the meeting. He dreaded the discussion. Emotions in these meetings tend to run high. Too often, it gets put off until the annual review, and then staff members are shocked when they don't receive the outstanding performance evaluation that they expected. For managers like Ray, staying on track with his key talking points and even rehearsing the conversation in advance with a mentor can be extremely helpful. William Gentry from the Center for Creative Leadership developed a three-step feedback model called the SBI (Situation–Behavior–Impact) to help manage these challenging conversations. [22]

STEP 1 – DESCRIBE THE SITUATION

In the case scenario above, Ray should refrain from discussing what the nurse may have done in other situations and stick to this particular staff meeting. He might open with – *"We are here to talk about what happened at the staff meeting last Thursday."*

STEP 2 – DESCRIBE THE BEHAVIOR

Ray would then next describe the actual, observable behavior being discussed. Keep to the facts. Don't insert opinions or judgments. He might say *"You interrupted me several times and raised your voice."* It is very important to keep it as specific as possible, not "you were very rude" which is open to interpretation.

STEP 3 – DESCRIBE THE IMPACT

Ray should then describe the effect that the behavior had both on him and the group. He might say, *"It might not have been your intent, but you interrupted the flow of the meeting and made it uncomfortable for me to continue with the agenda."*

NEXT STEPS

It is then essential to move into the next phase of the conversation where you acknowledge what the individual brings to the team. The manager might say, *"I am giving you these comments because you are a valued member of this team and I depend on your support – What can we do to fix this?"* Helping this nurse to come up with a different strategy to manage her concerns (other than being passive aggressive) can help to establish a plan moving forward.

When you see an improvement in behavior, reinforce it. This strategy may not work in all cases, but it is a good starting point and gives the employee the benefit of the doubt regarding their intent. For feedback to be useful, it has to have three components:

1. It is timely, so the recipient is clear on what the problem is.
2. It addresses one discreet behavior, so the recipient knows what to correct.
3. It provides clear guidance, so the recipient knows what they need to do to course correct.

Giving constructive feedback is not an innate skill. It takes practice and thoughtful reflection before you begin the conversation. It is helpful to have some go-to phrases that you use in giving staff feedback to guide your conversations such as the following statements: [23]

- I am having trouble understanding what happened here. Can you explain that to me?
- I'm concerned, and I want to hear from you what is going on from your perspective.
- It might not be your intent, but this is the way that your (actions or behaviors) were perceived.
- I can see what you were trying to accomplish. How could you have done this differently?
- What do you need from me to help you be more successful?

You should let your staff know in advance that you will be giving them feedback and even encourage them to ask for it proactively. Never give feedback when you are angry. Think intentionally about any crucial conversations that you need to have with staff members. Providing good feedback is an art that takes practice. The goal is to stay calm, stay positive and remain focused so that the message is received and the feedback does not fail.

MANAGING DIFFICULT STAFF BEHAVIORS

Learning how to deal with difficult personalities comes with the responsibilities of being a leader. As one of my mentors once told me, you will never enjoy these interactions, but over time, you will develop a thicker skin and learn how to manage them. We can all be difficult at times. The difference with difficult people is that they do it more often. It becomes a pattern of behavior. They may have been given feedback about their behavior, but have not made a consistent change. Part of what motivates difficult people is that they are often able to wear people down and get what they want. You may not be able to change the behavior of the difficult person, but you can change how you respond to it. By learning to disengage effectively, you will avoid getting hooked into the difficult behavior cycle.

DIFFICULT PERSONALITIES TYPES

Dr. Louellen Essex had identified the following four types of difficult personalities: [24]

- **The Volcano** – These individuals are abrupt, intimidating, domineering, arrogant, prone to personal attacks and extremely aggressive in their approach to getting what they want.

- **The Sniper** – These individuals are highly skilled in passive-aggressive behavior, take pot shots, engage in non-playful teasing, are mean-spirited and work to sabotage leaders.
- **The Chronic Complainer** – These individuals are whiny, find fault in every situation, accuse and blame others for problems, are self-righteous and see it as their responsibility to complain to set things right.
- **The Clam** – These individuals are disengaged, unresponsive, close down when you try to have a conversation, avoid answering direct questions and don't participate as members of the team.

TIPS FOR DEALING WITH DIFFICULT PEOPLE

You can probably identify the personality types of some of the difficult people you deal with from the list above. The more significant challenge is how you respond to the behavior. The following are some tips: [25]

1. **Don't try to change them** – Generally with difficult people; you are experiencing well-established patterns of behavior. Any change in behavior with a difficult person will only come if they take accountability for it. You can point out the behavior, but it is not your responsibility to change it.
2. **Don't take it personally** – The behaviors that you witness from difficult people are more a reflection of where they are personally than anything you may have said or done. They may be sick, tired or have extreme emotional problems. When you see an explosive reaction to a minor situation, you can be sure that the person is experiencing strong underlying emotions.
3. **Set boundaries** – Let the person know that you will respect them but expect to be treated with respect in return. Don't

tolerate yelling, and if necessary, tell the person that you need to remove yourself from the situation.

4. **Acknowledge their feelings** – You may not agree with their point of view but acknowledge that they appear to be very angry about a situation.

5. **Try empathy** – Recognize that it must be difficult to be stuck in a place of negativity or anger. Empathy can sometimes help to de-escalate explosive situations.

6. **Hold your ground** – Remember that you teach other people how to treat you so don't open the door to challenges.

7. **Use fewer words** – Less conversation is often more effective with difficult people. Use short, concise messages to drive your point home and set a time limit for how much you will engage in the discussion. Avoid using the word "attitude" because this will be viewed as very subjective, focus instead on the behavior.

While these tips are not guaranteed to work every time, you may find them helpful in many situations. The real key to managing difficult people is managing your reaction to the situation. In the end, the only behavior that you can truly control is your own.

REMEMBER

✓ Ideas about performance management have changed as younger generations in the workforce seek more feedback about how they are doing.

✓ Giving good feedback is an art that takes practice.

✓ The SBI (Situation–Behavior–Impact) framework is helpful to manage challenging conversations

✓ You cannot control the behavior of difficult people, but you can manage your own reaction.

CHAPTER 11

SELECT AND RETAIN THE RIGHT TEAM MEMBERS

M any parts of the US and other developed countries are experiencing severe nursing shortages. This is a significant change from a decade ago when turnover was low and new graduates often had challenges finding that first job. Today, the average RN vacancy rate in the US is 8.2%. Turnover ranges between 15 and 20% in many organizations. [26] Much of this nursing turnover occurs in the first three years of practice. [27] The replacement cost for an RN was recently estimated at an average of $49,500 with higher costs in specialty areas such as critical care and perioperative nursing. [28]

As a nurse leader coach, selecting and then retaining the right team members has never mattered more. Nurse managers are the chief recruitment and retention officers for their units. The evidence indicates that while nurses choose to be employed in organizations for what they have to offer, their reasons for leaving are usually because of challenges with their manager.

We know from a wide range of research studies that the relationship with one's immediate supervisor plays a critical role in satisfaction and retention. Research done by the Gallup corporation indicates that the four most valued qualities in leaders are trustworthiness, compassion, stability and the ability to foster hope. [5] Although these qualities matter, an important question is what specific behaviors leaders demonstrate that lead to higher levels of staff satisfaction and retention. A recent study helped to identify the characteristics of nurse leaders that contribute to nursing satisfaction. [29] These included the following findings:

THE LEADER EMPOWERS STAFF AND USES REFLECTIVE PRACTICE STRATEGIES TO ENHANCE NURSE AUTONOMY.
RNs identified empowerment as a critical leadership behavior – leaders must delegate decisions and trust staff. When a staff member makes a decision, they appreciate a leader who uses reflective practice strategies in a nonjudgmental way to assess outcomes.

THE LEADER IS VISIBLE AND PROMOTES INTERPERSONAL CONNECTIONS IN A SAFE AND CARING ENVIRONMENT.
RNs on units with high satisfaction report that their directors are visible, are accessible and look for ways to connect to staff. They take an interest in each of their nurses both professionally and personally. They use a strengths-based leadership approach to assess opportunities to promote development. They make sure that their staff is doing okay.

THE LEADER DEMONSTRATES PASSION AND VISION TO FOSTER A QUEST FOR EXCELLENCE.
Leaders who have high rates of staff satisfaction on their units are passionate about their work and their passion for excellence is contagious. They are transparent in sharing data as a way of looking for ways to improve.

THE LEADER MODELS' HIGH EXPECTATIONS AND PROFESSIONAL BEHAVIORS FOR STAFF.

Nurse leaders in units with high RN satisfaction lead by example. They are professional in how they look, speak and behave. They work hard to control their stress levels. They expect their nurses to be certified and give regular feedback on professional performance.

This study has significant findings for nurse leaders. Drilling down on key behaviors that matter in nursing leadership is critical to both select and retain great nurses.

SELECTING THE RIGHT STAFF

When vacancies climb on a unit, leaders may be tempted to fill positions with candidates that are not ideal. This rarely works out well. Sandy learned this lesson the hard way. She manages a busy ED in an inner-city safety net hospital. Her unit has been a revolving door of new staff who come and then stay only short periods of time. Sandy recognizes that part of the problem is the way she has approached recruitment. Sandy has not given it her full attention. Because of her high vacancy rates, she has hired candidates that she felt might not be a good fit for her unit. She has not taken the time to create a good strategy to market some of the important things that the unit could offer to good candidates. She also has not taken the time to develop performance or behavioral-based questions to get a sense of how the potential recruit might manage specific situations.

Sandy realized that she needed to be much more intentional in how she managed recruitment interviews. She developed a new strategy which included establishing an interview checklist that included the following items:

- Review the resume and application thoroughly before the interview.

- Meet the candidate in the lobby and walk him/her to the unit.
- Begin the interview by asking why the candidate was applying for a position in the ED.
- Ask the same performance-based questions of each nurse candidate.
- Explain the pros and cons of working in a safety-net facility with limited resources.
- Ask candidates about their career goals and explain her style of leadership coaching.
- Have the unit charge nurse give the candidate a tour of the unit and an opportunity to meet the staff.
- Describe the follow-up selection process and provide the candidate with her business card.
- Develop a welcome letter to the unit and include a new hire packet with the job description, the organizational mission, vision and values along with other essential information.

KEY FACTORS TO ASSESS

Many factors should be considered when evaluating candidates for hire. For Sally some of the key elements that she wanted to consider included the following:

- Education, work history and experience.
- Current knowledge, skills, and abilities relative to the needs of the unit.
- Cultural fit with the mission, vision, and values of the organization and team.
- Current staff competency skill mix.
- Interpersonal skills and questions asked.
- Professionalism, enthusiasm, and passion for the work.
- Patient advocacy and customer service.

- Professionalism and potential to contribute.
- Level of due diligence done by the candidate on the organization and specialty area.

PERFORMANCE-BASED INTERVIEWING

Performance-based or behavioral interviewing is an evidence-based method of interviewing staff. It involves giving candidates scenarios to assess their skills or open-ended questions about how they have managed specific situations in previous jobs. These answers provide insight into what you can expect in the future. The questions focus on learning how a candidate has performed in the past in a situation or on a task, the actions taken by them, and the outcomes of their decisions. They are also designed to help you assess the critical thinking skills of applicants. To create an effective interview instrument, examine the essential competencies expected in the position. Ask 2-3 questions for each competency and evaluate candidates on a sliding scale (1–a skill not evident to 4–strong evidence of skill) based on their responses. Examples of performance-based questions would include:

- Describe a situation in which you had to use your communication skills to de-escalate a situation with an angry patient. How did you manage the communication? How did you determine your message was received?
- Describe a time when you took personal accountability for conflict and initiated contact with the individual(s) involved to explain your actions. What steps did you take? What was the result?
- You have just received your assignment of five patients from the charge nurse. Walk me through how you would establish your priorities for the next hour.

- Share with me an example of an important personal goal that you set, and explain how you accomplished it.

Remember that interviewing is a two-way street so invite questions. As a manager, you should meet every candidate and ask about their expectations of you as their leader.

ONBOARDING STAFF

The successful hiring of great candidates is only the first step. New staff retention begins with proper onboarding. Dissatisfaction with employment often starts when a staff member receives a poor orientation to the unit. This is when your coaching for both performance and professional development needs to begin.

You should have regular check-ins scheduled at the end of the first week. Examples of questions to ask on check-in include the following:

1. Has our team made you feel welcome?
2. Did you receive what you needed to begin work? (new employee benefits information, ID badge, keys, email, and EMR access)
3. Do you have questions that have not been answered?
4. What challenges do you see in your new role?
5. Is there anything we should change to help new staff better adjust to the unit?

Nurse managers often delegate these responsibilities to preceptors or unit educators sometimes without good follow-up. That happened to Ray. He thought things were going smoothly with orientation on the unit he managed but then received feedback that there were issues with onboarding. New graduates received a thorough orientation as part of their residency, but the transition for more experienced nurses was hit and miss depending on the unit workload. He interviewed several recent new nurse hires and received valuable feedback about critical elements that seemed to be missing from orientation. He recognized that as a nurse leader coach, he too had a role in the process. Some steps that he could initiate to improve onboarding included the following:

A. BECOME MORE INTENTIONAL ABOUT HOW NEW STAFF IS WELCOMED AS AN IMPORTANT ADDITION TO THE UNIT.

When new staff joins your community, they have no history and may not be aware of important cultural norms, values, and behaviors. It is essential for the nurse leader coach to make sure they are welcomed and introduced to others as a valued team member. Preceptors play a vital role in the onboarding of new staff and should be carefully selected to make sure they are positive role models. New staff should be encouraged to ask questions and contact you directly with any concerns that they may have.

B. ENSURE NEW STAFF RECEIVE A THOROUGH ORIENTATION EVEN IF THEY ARE EXPERIENCED.

New staff should receive orientation at both the hospital and unit level. Key policies and procedures should be reviewed. A thorough orientation checklist provided by either the manager or unit educator should be used to ensure that all new staff receives the same information. Don't skip steps even when you are short staffed. Always remember, you are setting the stage during orientation for a smooth transition.

C. DO REGULAR CHECK-INS ON THE PROGRESS OF NEW STAFF MEMBERS.

Nurse managers should schedule a meeting with new staff at the end of the first week, at the 30-day point, at 60 days and mid-year to see how things are progressing and to assess satisfaction with employment. This is an excellent time to assess whether expectations are being met, answer questions, clarify policies, evaluate challenges and use the information to refine the onboarding process.

D. BEGIN THE PROFESSIONAL DEVELOPMENT COACHING PROCESS.

The late Dr. Stephen Covey in *The 7 Habits of Highly Effective People,* advised that we should begin with the end in mind. [30] This is good advice in coaching new staff. Much of the first six months of employment is usually spent on performance coaching, but long-term commitment will be built if you include professional development coaching. Learn about each new staff member's personal goals for their career and begin the individual development plan. Help staff to establish at least two to three personal development goals. The goals should include actions and a timeline. Every manager should have a list of professional growth opportunities available to staff on their unit such as:

- Certification preparation classes
- Cross-departmental committee participation
- New graduate mentorship
- Charge nurse classes
- Unit practice council participation
- Community leadership activities (heart walk, United Way drive, mission trips)

REDUCING TURNOVER

After almost of decade of low nursing turnover rates, many health systems are once again experiencing high rates of nursing turnover. [26,28] With an improved economy, many Baby Boomers who had put off retirement, are now leaving. New staff members can find many more employment options and are willing to leave if dissatisfied. Some turnover is to be expected, however when it climbs above 10%, there are high costs in salary replacement, training of new staff and potential quality issues. Depending on the specialty area, the cost of an RN loss can reach $82,000. If you have 500 RN FTE and 17.9% leave each year – you could experience a revenue loss of as much as 7.4 million dollars a year. Karlene Kerfoot, the Chief Nursing Officer for GE Healthcare, recommends the following four strategies to reduce nurse turnover: [31]

1. **Minimize Overtime Expectations** – Mandatory overtime or on call requirements are huge dissatisfiers especially for Millennial nurses who value their time off. Once staffing problems start, it can be a vicious cycle as leaders try to safely staff units by requiring staff to work more hours.

2. **Practice Shared Governance** – Lack of empowerment and involvement in decision making leads to disengagement. Shared governance is one strategy to try to keep staff involved in decision making. This also requires nurse leaders who value shared governance and practice at the unit level. Leadership research consistently shows that the quality of the relationship that a nurse has with his/her manager is a strong predictor of retention.

3. **Implement Data Driven Staffing** – Inadequate staffing is a frequently cited reason why nurses are leaving employers today. With skill mixes trending toward less experienced nurses, this is especially important to provide the level of support that is needed. Nurses may be more likely to leave if they are placed in patient care situations that they are not equipped to handle.

4. **Develop Quality of Life Initiatives** – The current healthcare environment is complex and often chaotic. Healthcare staff is at high risk for burnout as expectations of patients and employers continue to increase. Quality of life initiatives that promote resiliency are essential today. This could include support for learning

meditation and mindfulness, quiet rooms, gym memberships, on-site childcare, yoga and more time off for family and friends. Actively promoting friendships at work matters because Gallup has considerable data to support that having a best friend at work is linked to retention and engagement.[5]

Preventing staff turnover is an ongoing challenge for nurse leaders. In an interesting book *When* about the science of timing, Daniel Pink provides fascinating insight about some of the drivers that lead to employee resignations.[32] Employment anniversary dates play a crucial role in decisions about seeking new employment. Pink advises that staff may often ask themselves whether they want to be in the organization the next year. Armed with this evidence, nurse leaders should consider keeping a list of employee's anniversary dates and planning proactive coaching conversations 90 days in advance of these dates.

Retaining New Graduates

The biggest challenges with staff retention are in the first three years of practice with turnover rates as high as 50%.[27] There are many reasons for difficulties in retaining new graduates, but a lack of leadership support has been identified as a critical factor in exit interview surveys. New graduates want their managers to be leader coaches. They may sometimes resist feedback or see it as criticism but will be more receptive if it is presented as a "coaching moment."

While reality shock has always been part of the new nurse transition, the transformation from student to nurse is even more challenging today. Good coaching can make a significant difference in both reducing the frustration felt by new graduates, and retaining them in their initial work settings. Some key approaches that managers can use to provide better support to new graduates include the following:

1. **Remember what it was like to be a novice**

   Experienced nurses move through their workday often giving little thought to their clinical decision-making process. Nursing responses that appear so evident to a seasoned nurse may not be as obvious for the newer nurse. New graduates are in the novice stage of their nursing development. They rely on following the recalled rules of practice that they learn in school and may not grasp the full context of a nursing situation. The novice nurse may appear to be slow in their actions and not focused on tasks that need to be immediately accomplished. This is part of the development on the continuum from novice to expert.

2. **Promote critical thinking skills**

   A frequent complaint about novice nurses is that they lack critical thinking skills. Good coaching is vital to the development of strong clinical reasoning. New nurses need to be provided with learning opportunities where a coach helps them through guided discussion and reflection to connect their thinking and action.

3. **Be sensitive to generational differences**

   When coaching novice nurses, it is essential to consider generational differences. With up to five generations (Veterans, Baby Boomers, Generation X, Millennials, Generation Z) in today's workplace, you may find yourself coaching a novice nurse who has very different attitudes, beliefs, work habits and experiences than your own. As the world changes, generational cohorts have different life experiences. These experiences create preferences about how a generation wants to be coached and motivated by those who work with them. Most new graduates entering the workforce today are Millennials (born between 1980 and 2000). Both the Millennials and Generation Z expect more coaching and regular feedback than other generations in the workplace. They are optimistic and goal oriented but also want structure, guidance and an extensive orientation.

4. GIVE THEM HOPE AND ENCOURAGEMENT

Having a unit culture that promotes the importance of coaching, learning and teaching will help to build the confidence of novice nurses. Today's health-care environments are often very chaotic. New graduates can quickly become overwhelmed and feel professionally isolated. The novice's sense of self-trust in their judgment is often tenuous. Hope and encouragement about the progress that they are making is critical feedback, especially when it comes from nurse leaders.

Coaching our novice nurses is a responsibility that all professionals in nursing share. Nurse managers need to build a culture that supports new graduates and encourages career growth.

UNDERSTANDING ORGANIZATIONAL LOYALTY

Historically, organizational loyalty was defined in terms of longevity when it was not unusual to work for one employer for decades. With the economic downturns that began in the 1980s, a lifetime commitment to one organization was no longer possible for many employees. Experienced, well-performing staff were often "right-sized" out of an organization through no fault of their own. Job tenure in all industries has become shorter. Both organizations and employees began to view commitment differently. Today, experts who study organizational suggest that there has been a redefinition.

Jeff, a Baby Boomer manager, is frustrated with the trend of shorter job tenures. He perceives his younger staff as being less loyal because they are more likely to leave the unit for career growth. His organization recently revised the unit transfer policy no longer requiring nurses to stay on their initial unit of assignment for one year before requesting a transfer. Jeff has been an outspoken critic of the new policy. His CNO showed him data that supported the change. When nurses were not allowed to transfer, they sought employment elsewhere. It was resulting in a loss of some of the best young nurses in the organization.

Jeff is not alone in his concern about the shifts that have taken place in thinking about organizational loyalty. There has been a significant increase in career mobility, and even a propensity to hypermobility. Loyalty has been redefined to mean aligning with the values and goals of the organization and giving one's best to an organization *while one is employed*. This may or may not involve a long-term commitment to the organization. The reality is that just because someone has worked for your organization for twenty years does not necessarily mean he or she is loyal or even engaged in his or her work.

INSPIRING ORGANIZATIONAL LOYALTY

Inspiring organizational loyalty is essential in healthcare and has been shown to result in better patient outcomes. Five strategies recommended by industry experts include:[33]

1. **Promote identification with the organization** – Help staff to see how the mission and values of the organization are consistent with his or her personal values.
2. **Connect staff to the success/status of the organization** – Encourage staff to develop a sense of pride in an organization by showing how their contributions matter in the organization's accomplishments and status.
3. **Create security** – Give staff a sense of security about their employability and potential career paths within the organization.

4. **Provide recognition and opportunities to build skills** – Validate the skills and worth of staff and promote camaraderie and teamwork. Most nursing staff today look for opportunities to develop their skills and mastery at their jobs. Mastery is a desire to get better at something that matters.

5. **Build trust** – build an environment of trust and transparency. Demonstrate that as a leader, you trust your staff and can personally be trusted.

It is true that organizational loyalty is more challenging, to achieve today. Yet, committed nurse leader coaches can help staff to identify with the goals of the organization, feel excited about their work, and promote a sense of belonging.

REMEMBER:

✓ We know from a wide range of research studies that the relationship with one's immediate supervisor plays a critical role in satisfaction and retention.

✓ Performance-based interviewing is an evidence-based approach to interviewing that involves giving candidates scenarios to assess their skills or open-ended questions about how they have managed specific situations in previous jobs.

✓ Dissatisfaction with employment often begins when staff members feel like they have been given a poor orientation to the unit.

✓ Both organizations and staff now view organizational loyalty and commitment differently.

CHAPTER 12

LEAD CHANGE

Today's healthcare environment is described as being characterized by volatility, uncertainty, complexity, and ambiguity. [34] The turmoil is an outcome of different forces all driven by rising health care costs. There is national pressure from policy experts and insurance payers aimed at healthcare providers and organizations to achieve greater efficiency, improve quality, and reduce costs. The value of care being delivered is now measured by a growing number of performance measures that impact both reimbursement and regulation. These forces have led to a continuous change in healthcare environments. Policies, practices, and technology are shifting at a pace that staff is finding challenging. Nurse leaders at the frontlines of care are being asked to drive changes that often meet resistance.

The pace of change is expected to continue. Coaching staff through the change process requires highly skilled leadership. We are often asking staff to make significant changes in their practice with new policies or initiatives. These changes are difficult because our practices are in essence a collection of habits. Charles Duhigg, an investigative reporter for the New York Times, has written an interesting evidence-based book about how habits are formed and what we can do to change them. [35]

Duhigg contends that habits make up 40% of our daily routines, whether at work or home. What you see in your work environments is in a sense a collection of habits that develop over time. Habits are the brain's way of saving energy. A mistake that leaders make is that they forget how ingrained habits are. Hardwiring a new habit can take more than the 30 days that we often devote to implementing new initiatives. This is why change can be so challenging. It is also the reason why experienced staff may have more challenges with change than novices.

Why Change Fails

Not all change is successful. Mary learned this lesson as a new leader in her unit. During her orientation to the role, she was advised that the policy for nursing shift report was that nurses should do it as part of bedside rounding. Although this change had been implemented more than two years ago at her new organization, it was not being done on her unit. She asked the staff about it and was told that bedside rounding did not work on the unit. The previous leader had given the okay to abandon the new policy. Mary decided that it was important to consider what went wrong before she began the practice again. She identified the following problems:

1. **Initiative fatigue in the organization** – At the time that bedside rounding was first introduced, there were many other new initiatives that followed. Staff began to see these changes as the flavor of the month.

2. **Lack of frontline leadership support** – While the initiative was an organizational requirement, Mary's predecessor was not fully committed to the initiative nor did she ensure adequate follow-up.

3. **Failure to engage staff in the planning** – The initiative was designed at the organizational level, and frontline staff on the unit were not involved with any of the planning.

4. **Poor planning** – There was a lack of detailed planning about how, where and when to initiate the change. There were no plans for evaluation.

5. **Failure to sustain the initiative over time** – While the initiative started reasonably well, it was never embedded into the culture of the unit, and there was no follow-up to sustain the effort across time.

STRATEGIES TO PROMOTE SUCCESS

Like many new managers, Mary learned how complicated it could be to both implement and sustain change even when it is an evidence-based practice. It will be important to consider strategies that will promote success when it is reintroduced. To be more successful the next time around, Mary will want to do the following:

1. *Create a Sense of Urgency* – To effectively implement a new initiative, staff in an organization need to understand why it is needed. You need to tell a compelling story of why change is required.

2. *Consider the Organizational Culture* – Successful initiatives from other organizations may not be directly transferable to an organization with a different culture. The unit culture needs to be carefully considered in the planning process.

3. ***Get Staff Buy-In*** – Staff, especially those serving in charge nurse roles need to have the opportunity to discuss their concerns about initiatives. Once the decision is made to move forward, staff need to be directly asked to commit to the success of the effort.

4. ***Involve Staff in Every Aspect of Planning*** – To create buy-in and develop a better plan; staff needs to be involved in the planning process. Select frontline staff champions that can help in the roll-out, training and evaluation process.

5. ***Don't Make Assumptions about Training Needs*** – Carefully plan how, when and where to educate staff about the initiative. A lecture may not be the right strategy when the change calls for new skills that need to be practiced and observed.

6. ***Plan an Ongoing Evaluation*** – To be successful; initiatives should become part of the culture. They need to become part of the organizational dashboard evaluation and remain a priority after the initial launch.

HELPING STAFF TO MANAGE CHANGE

Not all of us accept change in the same way or on the same timeline. It is essential to meet people where they are in the change process. Accept that some people will not be as far along as you might want them to be. Where they are in the process will depend on their comfort with change (ability to take on new learning) and capacity for change (ability to learn that which is required). Change can be quite emotional. It often means letting go of something that you have valued in the past. Where people are in the acceptance process can be very variable, and leaders need to assess this with their staff.

Staff depends on their leaders to help them understand the meaning of the changes that are discussed. How leaders use language to frame people, situations, and events has significant consequences for the way individuals make sense of the world and leadership actions. Most nursing staff understand that the costs, fragmentation in care and variable outcomes in today's system are not sustainable moving into the future.

You will observe different patterns in how staff response to change. Kerry Bunker suggests that there are four distinct response to change (*entrenched, overwhelmed, poser or learner*).[36] Entrenched staff may decide that they outlast change or maybe it won't happen until they retire. Overwhelmed staff have high anxiety levels and may have feelings of depression or powerlessness. Posers exhibit a high level of confidence in their ability to deal with changes but may not have the self-awareness and actual competence that they need. Learners feel challenged and stretched but are determined to move forward. They seek learning opportunities to expand their skills in response to the change. Learners can be a leader's best allies in helping other staff transition during changes.

In most situations where we are asked to change, we are substituting the old for the new and unfamiliar. This can make us feel insecure about our work and is often personally exhausting. The response of leaders to change or turbulence has a powerful effect on their staff. There are always possibilities in change that can lead to a new, brighter future, and this needs to be conveyed. Leaders who remain calm, truthful and optimistic in their communications help to prevent the spread of misinformation and reduce staff anxiety. There are silver linings in any situation, and the leader needs to be the first to help everyone see what those are. An optimistic attitude and outlook on the part of the leader can be very energizing and contagious. It will motivate your staff to do their best. You need to expect success if you are to achieve it.

TIMING IN LEADERSHIP

Great ideas and initiatives can and do fail if leaders try to push change at a time when it is not right for the organization. Strategic priorities and key staff can quickly shift in today's environment. John Maxwell identified the law of timing as one of his *21 Irrefutable Laws of Leadership.*[37] He observed that timing is often the difference between success and failure in an endeavor or in dealing with a staff issue. Developing a good sense of timing in your work is a vital nursing leadership strategy in managing change. Some key questions to ask yourself include the following:

1. **DO I HAVE A GOOD GRASP OF THE ORGANIZATIONAL CLIMATE?**
   Sometimes the organizational climate may not be ready for new initiatives or change. I once visited with a new chief nursing officer in a small rural hospital. She had identified many professional practice issues that need to be corrected but observed, *"I have to pace what I do here. Change needs to be implemented more slowly than I would like but it is the culture."* Astute nurse leaders carefully study their organizational cultures and are not tone deaf to what is happening in their environment.

2. **WHAT ARE THE COMPETING FACTORS THAT COULD INFLUENCE SUCCESS?**
   Sometimes great ideas cannot gain traction in organizations, because there are too many competing factors in the environment. It is important to explore what these competing factors are.

3. **DO I HAVE THE EXPERIENCE TO LAUNCH THIS INITIATIVE AND THE CONFIDENCE OF THOSE WHO WILL BE IMPACTED?**
   It is often said that the right action at the right time by the right leader can result in incredible success. There are times as a leader when you need to decide whether you are the right person to accept a specific leadership role, drive a change in an organization or implement a new project. The answer could be yes, but it may also be no.

4. Have I created the conditions for success?

Projects sometimes fail because of inadequate preparation. As a leader, you may need to delay an initiative until you are sure that you have set your team up for success.

5. Have I carefully listened to my intuition about timing?

Leaders are often very excited about their initiatives but sometimes know in their gut that there are problems. Seeking Magnet ™ designation presents an interesting dilemma for some nurse leaders. Several chief nursing officers that I know have put the brakes on their Magnet applications because they felt from a timing standpoint, the organization was just not ready. This required leadership courage but wise leaders learn to listen to their intuition.

Successful leaders are good planners who understand that the building blocks need to be in place for initiatives to succeed. Leadership is critical at every stage of the change process. We can't let up. We need to implement tools to measure our progress. Nurse leaders sometimes complain about lack of staff compliance yet the problem is that we don't build in mechanisms to hardwire changes into practice. Nurse leader coaches know that they also must create a culture that reinforces the new habit to make it stick and this includes changing rewards and recognition to influence the development of new behaviors. It is only through the intentional evaluation of whether the change is working that success can be achieved.

REMEMBER:

✓ Coaching staff through the change process requires highly skilled leadership.

✓ Hardwiring a new habit can take more than the 30 days that we often devote to implementing new initiatives.

✓ It is essential to meet people where they are in the change process.

✓ Successful leaders are good planners who understand that the building blocks need to be in place for initiatives to succeed.

References – Part 2

1. Gallup Corporation. *State of the American Workplace 2017.* Available at https://news.gallup.com/reports/199961/state-american-workplace-report-2017.aspx. Accessed July 27th, 2018.
2. Virkstis K. The national prescription for nurse engagment: Best practices for enfranchising frontline staff in transformation. *Nurse Advisory Board Research Report.* April 10th, 2014. Available at https://www.advisory.com/research/nursing-executive-center/studies/2014/national-prescription-for-nurse-engagement Accessed August 2nd, 2018.
3. Hess V. *6 Shortcuts to Employee Engagement: Lead and Succeed in a Do-More-With-Less World.* Catalyst Consulting LLC; 2013.
4. Robinson J. Outcome based managers focus on people and the finish line. *Gallup Business Journal.* June 21, 2018. Available at https://www.gallup.com/workplace/235961/outcome-based-managers-focus-people-finish-line.aspx Accessed August 2nd, 2018.
5. Gallup. *First Break all the Rules: What the World's Greatest Managers do Differently.* New York: Gallup Press; 2016.

6. Gordon J. *The Energy Bus: Ten Rules to fuel you Life, Work and Team with Positive Energy.* New Jersey: Wiley & Sons; 2007.

7. Rath T, Conchie B. *Strengths-Based Leadership.* New York: Gallup Press; 2008.

8. Rath T. *Strengths Finder 2.0.* New York: Gallup Press; 2007.

9. Goldsmith M, Reiter M. *Triggers: Creating Behavior that Lasts – Becoming the Person You Want to Be.* New York: Crown; 2015.

10. Gentry, W.A. and the Center for Creative Leadership (2016). *Be the boss everyone wants to work for: A guide for new leaders.* Oakland, CA: Berrett-Koehler Publishers.

11. Bungay-Stanier M. *The Coaching Habit: Say Less, Ask More and Change the Way You Lead Forever.* Toronto: Box of Crayons; 2016.

12. Ross, J. (May 6th, 2009 HBR Blog) How to ask better questions. Available at https://hbr.org/2009/05/real-leaders-ask.html. Accessed August 2nd, 2018.

13. Sinek S. *Start with Shy: How Great Leaders Inspire Everyone to Take Action.* New York: Portfolio Press; 2011.

14. Agency for Healthcare Research and Quality. (b). *TeamSTEPPS* Available at https://www.ahrq.gov/teamstepps/index.html Accessed August 2nd, 2018.

15. Hefferman, M. (May 20th, 2013 CBS Money Watch Blog). How do leaders respond to email? Available at https://www.cbsnews.com/news/how-do-leaders-respond-to-email/ Accessed August 2nd, 2018.

16. Simmons A. *The Story Factor: Inspiration, Influence and Persuasion through the Art of Story Telling.* New York: Perseus Publishing; 2001.

17. Kimann T. The conflict mode iinstrument. Available at http://www.kilmanndiagnostics.com/overview-thomas-kilmann-conflict-mode-instrument-tki

18. Augsburger, D. *Caring Enough to Ccnfront.* Ventura, CA: Regal Publications; 1981.

19. Sherman, R.O. Carefronting, *American Nurse Today, 7*(10), 72-74; 2012.

20. Sharpe, D. & Johnson, E. *Managing Conflict with Your Boss.* Greensboro, NC: Center for Creative Leadership; 2002.

21. Dyess S. & Sherman RO. The first year of practice: New graduate learning needs and transition experiences. *Journal of Continuing Education in Nursing. 40*(9), 403-409; 2009.

22. Gentry W. *Be the boss everyone wants to work for: A guide for new leaders.* Oakland CA: Berrett-Koehler Publishers; 2016.

23. Blatcheley A. Giving feedback: A guide for nurse managers. *Nurse Leader* .15(5) 331-334; 2017.

24. Louellen Essex and Associates. *Dealing with Difficult People in the Healthcare Setting.* 2006 Available at http://www.louellenessex.com/pdf/DealingwithDifficultPeopleWorkbook.pdf

25. Sherman RO. Managing difficult people. *The American Nurse Today.* 8(7), 40-42; 2013.

26. ANM Healthcare. (2018b). *Worsening shortages and growing consequences: CNO survey on nurse supply and demand.* Accessed at https://www.amnhealthcare.com/cno-survey on-supply-demand/

27. Kovner C T, Djukic M, Fatehi F K, Fletcher J, Jun J, Brewer C., Chacko, T. Estimating and preventing hospital internal turnover of newly licensed nurses: A panel survey. *International Journal of Nursing Studies, 60,* 251-262; 2016.

28. NSI. 2018 National health care retention and RN staffing report. Accessed at http://www.nsinursingsolutions.com/Files/assets/library/retention institute/NationalHealthcareRNRetentionReport2018.pdf

29. Burke D., Flanagan, J., Ditomassi, M. & Hickey, P.A. Characteristics of Nurse Directors that Contribute to Registered Nurse Satisfaction. *Journal of Nursing Administration. 47*(4), 219-225; 2017.

30. Covey S. *The 7 Habits of Highly Successful People.* New York: Simon & Schuster; 1989.

31. Kefoot K. *Four measures that are key to retaining nurses.* 2015. Accessed at https://www.hhnmag.com/articles/3253-four-measures-that-are-key-to-retaining-nurses

32. Pink DH. *When: The Scientific Secrets of Perfect Timing.* New York: Riverhead Books; 2018.

33. Robinson S. *Fierce Loyalty: Unlocking the DNA of Wildly Successful Communities.* London: Hayfield Publishing; 2012.

34. Escobeda, M. (December 3, 2015). Leading change in a VUCA world. Accessed at http://www.jhartfound.org/blog/leading-change-in-a-vuca-world/

35. Duhigg, C. *The Power of Habit: Why We do What We do in Life and Business.* New York: Random House; 2012.

36. Bunker K A. In Rush. S. (Editor) *On Leading in Times of Change.* Greensboro, N.C.: Center for Creative Leadership; 2012

37. Maxwell J C. *The 21 Irrefutable Laws of Leadership.* Nashville: Thomas Nelson Publishers; 2007.

PART 3

COACHING TEAMS TO HIGHER PERFORMANCE

"Talent wins games, but teamwork and
intelligence win championships."

MICHAEL JORDAN

CHAPTER 13

FOSTER EFFECTIVE TEAMWORK

I n the first two parts of this book, our focus has been on building a coaching foundation and developing your coaching skills. In our final section, we examine how to effectively coach teams to a higher level of performance. Casey Stengel, the beloved manager of many major league baseball teams, once noted that *"Finding good players is easy. Getting them to play as a team is another story."* The same could be said of teams in healthcare settings. High-performance work teams in any environment rarely occur naturally. They must be created and coached. Guiding team members to get past their day to day problems, conflicts and communication issues toward a goal of working as a high-performance work team is a significant leadership challenge. Nowhere are the stakes higher than in the healthcare, where team synergy and interdependence are required for high quality patient outcomes.

If you have worked on a highly effective and smooth-running team, it is an experience you are not likely to forget. Effective teams have the following ten key characteristics: [1]

1. Clear goals that everyone on the team works towards
2. Clarity about the role and contributions of each team member
3. Open and clear communication
4. Effective decision making
5. Engaged team members in the work of the team
6. Appreciation of diversity – generational, cultural and diversity in thinking
7. Effective management of conflicts
8. Trust among team members
9. Cooperative relationships
10. Participative leadership

Leaders play a crucial role in helping a team to develop the ability to collaborate effectively, build relationships and trust, innovate and achieve results at a consistently high level. They must also create environments where there is a willingness to assist other team members in their work sometimes referred to as *team backup*. [2] To do this, the leader must know their team members, and understand their strengths and how to motivate them. It all begins with setting the stage for quality communication among team members.

Attention must be paid to establishing venues in which these conversations can take place whether they occur in team briefings, meetings or at social events. There needs to be a zone of safety created at meetings where team members can constructively challenge current processes, procedures or how the team is functioning. Team ground rules are critical to developing strong relationships and trust.

Team members need to understand that they are expected to respect one another, listen to each other, care for each other, accept responsibility for their behavior and learn from each other, which helps to foster a sense of commitment. A good coaching exercise is to ask team members to assess how well the team is doing. Members can be asked how accurate the following statements are for their team: [3]

- The goals of our team are clearly stated and known by members.
- The members of our team are committed to accomplishing our shared team goals.
- Our team accomplishes its goals.
- The talents of each of our team members are fully utilized.
- Each member of the team fulfills the role he or she is expected to play.
- Our team deals with conflict in an effective manner.

The collective answers to a team assessment can be a powerful way to introduce team building initiatives that build on a team's strengths and addresses weaknesses. Tim tried this assessment with his perioperative staff assigned to the orthopedic team. He had received feedback that the nurses on the team did not work well together but wanted concrete data before he addressed the issue. Using a five-point Likert scale with response options from 1 (this rarely happens on our team) to 5 (this always happens on our team), the average overall score given by staff in response to the six questions was 12 out of a possible 30. He was not surprised to see these low scores, and it provided him with a framework to begin team building. He clearly understands that teamwork is at the heart of all great achievement. Teams members offer valuable perspectives and strengths in meeting the needs of patients that are broader and deeper than that of any one individual.

TEAM BUILDING

As Tim learned, building successful teams requires involvement by the leader. He recognized that he had not done an effective job of setting leadership expectations about how the team would function. This is a critical step in team building. Without it, individual egos, insecurities and personal beliefs can get in the way of goal achievement. Participation on and contributing to a team cannot be optional behavior. Backing up other team members needs to be an expectation. As their leader, he needed to be crystal clear about team goals, behavioral expectations of each team member and the consequences of toxic behaviors. These are building blocks for team accountability. The situation with Tim's team had reached a crisis point because he had not provided the ongoing coaching and feedback that teams need to sustain performance and manage conflict. This team also lacked the ground rules or norms required to ensure efficiency and success. Tim's rebuilding efforts included the following steps:

1. Establish a clear purpose for the work that all team members can agree on.
2. Promote shared decision making and accountability to achieve team goals.
3. Foster mechanisms to open communication and resolve conflicts on the team.
4. Clarify the role, value, and assignment of each team member.
5. Build team behavioral norms and shared values.

Team building is one of the most important responsibilities a manager has. It is not a one and done activity but rather a journey that never ends. As new members join the team, they need to be encouraged to participate in building the team culture. Current team members may need to be encouraged to be nurturing of novices and see their development as part of a professional legacy. To create high-performance work teams, reward and recognition programs need to include awards for team achievement. Team recognition programs help to build team esteem and send a strong message that effective teamwork matters.

MANAGING MULTIGENERATIONAL TEAMS

Today's healthcare teams are diverse. It is not uncommon to have up to five generations working together. This was Sherry's experience. She has been in her role as trauma ICU manager for 17 years. When she was initially appointed to the role, she adopted an approach in her leadership that felt comfortable for her. Over the years, she noticed her team had changed and was now comprised of more generational groups. Some of the leadership strategies that had worked well for her in the past were no longer effective. She took the time to study the generational literature and to use what she learned in managing her team. She found that the communication needs of staff were different. Her seasoned nurses, many of whom were Baby Boomers, wanted to come to her office and have a conversation. Her Millennial and Gen Z nurses preferred texting their questions, and expected immediate answers. She stopped trying to impose her communication preferences and values. Sherry recognized that she needed to flex her leadership if she was to be effective in leading a multi-generational team. A one size fits all approach would not work. She had taken the time to learn about generational differences to more effectively coach her staff. One the recommendations in the literature was to use the evidence-based **ACORN** framework described below in her coaching:[4]

Accommodate Differences – You need to take the time to know your staff as individuals, and learn what is important to them. When possible, make an effort to accommodate their personal scheduling needs, work-life balance issues and non-traditional life-styles. Recognize that each generation has different ideas about communication styles, career planning, and how they would like to be recognized and rewarded.

Create Workplace Choices – The workplace should be shaped around the work being done, the customers being served and the people who work there. Shorten the chain of command and reduce bureaucracy. Create a relaxed and informal work environment with lots of humor and connectedness.

Operate with a Sophisticated Management Style – Nurses today look for transformational leaders who provide clear vision and direction to the work. Leaders should give feedback, offer rewards and recognition as appropriate, and avoid micromanagement. Every generational cohort wants to be respected and fairly treated. Leaders should strive to be perceived as fair, inclusive, and a good communicator.

Respect Competence and Initiative – Assume the best of your employees. Treat everyone, from the newest recruit to the most seasoned employee, as if they have great things to offer. Seek to maximize the strengths of your staff instead of focusing on weaknesses. Take time to hire the right people. Find out what motivates each of your staff members and work hard to keep them engaged.

Nourish retention – Nurse leaders matter when it comes to retention because nurses don't leave organizations but rather leaders. Each generation has different expectations of their leaders. In the book *Workplace 2020*, researchers highlight some differences.[5] The Veteran cohort's #1 trait that they look for in a manager is someone who will work well across the different generational groups. Baby Boomers look for leaders who will give them straight feedback. Both the Millennials and Generation Z want leaders who will coach them, and help them to develop their careers.

The ACORN imperatives seem simple and straightforward, yet not all nurse leaders take the time to practice them. It is easy to get blinded by your generational values and fight the need to flex your management style. Implementing the ACORN principles takes work and a different way of looking at how to manage multiple generations. However, the rewards are immense.

AVOID GROUP THINK

Group Think has been defined as a psychological phenomenon that occurs within a group of people when the desire for harmony or conformity in the group results in an incorrect or flawed decision-making outcome. Group members try to minimize conflict and reach a consensus decision without critical evaluation of alternative ideas or viewpoints, and by isolating themselves from outside influences. In situations where there is group think, loyalty to the group way of thinking pressures individuals to avoid raising controversial issues or alternative solutions. When this occurs, there is a loss of individual creativity and independent thinking.

An often-cited example of group think is the Challenger spaceship disaster. Before the launch, some engineers on the project raised concerns about the ability of the O-ring seals to withstand the launch temperatures and opposed the launch. They were pressured by the group to reconsider their position and reverse their initial no-go position which they did with disastrous results. Although this is an extreme example, you can probably think of cases in your setting. Jack saw this in a strategic planning session that he participated in with other leaders from his health system. There was groupthink about plans to build a freestanding ER. There were a few in the group like Jack who felt that this was not a wise idea for solid reasons including the proximity to a highly regarded hospital. Their views were quickly over-ruled and not carefully considered in this groupthink situation. The decision ultimately turned out to be an expensive failure for the organization.

Leaders can prevent groupthink situations by coaching team members to appreciate diverse viewpoints. The following is advice from the experts:[6]

- Establish group norms to actively encourage and promote divergent thinking.
- Actively seek and value age, cultural, educational and ideas-related diversity on teams.
- Ask whether there is a different perspective on the issue being discussed by the team.
- Reward truth speakers by acknowledging their contributions to the discussion.
- Don't voice an opinion as the leader until you have sought the viewpoints of all team members.
- Embrace conflict, don't quell it in the interest of harmony.
- Before making a major decision, go around the room and ask each member for the pros and cons of the decision.

As a nurse leader, it is important to remember that groupthink has benefits in some situations. When the work involves a large team, it can allow the group to make decisions, complete tasks, and finish projects more quickly and efficiently. However, this phenomenon comes with costs that need to be considered.

REMEMBER

✓ High-performance work teams in any setting rarely occur naturally. They must be created and coached.

✓ Team ground rules are critical to developing strong relationships and trust.

✓ Today's healthcare teams are diverse in composition, and a one size fits all leadership style does not work.

✓ Leaders can prevent groupthink situations by coaching team members to appreciate diverse viewpoints.

CHAPTER 14

Promote Interprofessional Teamwork

Healthcare has been described as a team sport because the contributions of each discipline are so interdependent. Quality healthcare outcomes only happen in environments where there is strong interprofessional teamwork. Having a team of experts does not necessarily mean that you have an expert team. Teamwork must be built. Getting interprofessional teams on the same page, or even together in the same place to communicate can be challenging. The concept of everyone being involved and participating is the key to effective interdisciplinary work. The stakes are high if this does not happen. Most medical errors involve breakdowns in communication among team members. Ineffective interprofessional teamwork is a patient safety issue, and some experts believe it is strongly correlated to higher patient mortality.

Nurse leader coaches need to create a culture that strongly values interprofessional teamwork. On interprofessional teams, decisions are reached collectively by the group. Involvement and participation in patient care decisions is the key to effective group functioning. Interprofessional teamwork requires individual involvement. Professionals cannot be allowed to opt out because given the opportunity, some will. This happened on Zoe's surgical unit. Her patient satisfaction scores involving communication with health providers were low. From her research, Zoe learned that interprofessional bedside rounding is an evidence-based strategy to improve the patient experience and communication. Her process to introduce the rounding was well thought out. Families and patients expressed appreciation for the opportunity to have all the team members together to discuss care. She was sure that customer service scores would improve over time. Then without notice or discussion, the rounds were discontinued because key physician team members complained to the CEO that it interfered with the pace of their work.

In thinking about why the rounding initiative had not worked, Zoe realized that she had not established a sense of urgency for the change. She realized that every discipline has a unique culture, language and a mental model in how they approach patient situations. This needs to be respected and listened to. Professional team members are often surprised by the knowledge and clinical abilities of other disciplines. This respect may not happen initially but does grow over time.

Zoey had failed to communicate the purpose of the initiative effectively. The outcomes she sought were better communication in care planning and stronger interdisciplinary teamwork. We sometimes assume that professionals will see the value in interdisciplinary collaboration without being explicit about the benefits. In the course of their training, providers tend to become socialized into their professions and subsequently develop negative biases and naïve perceptions of the roles of other members of the health care team. To practice effectively in an interprofessional primary health care team, however, one must have a clear understanding of other members' unique contributions, their educational backgrounds, areas of high achievement, and limitations.

Changing Mental Models

The promotion of interprofessional teamwork may involve changing current mental models about how care is delivered, and the value of expertise brought by other interprofessional team members. Nurse leaders often need to help professionals see the value in collective knowledge and talents by explicitly soliciting these viewpoints on patient situations when planning care for patients.

A common issue in interprofessional teamwork is the problem of "turf battles. These struggles over protecting the scope and authority of a profession involve issues of autonomy, accountability, and identity. Team members may be reluctant to take advice or suggestions from members of other disciplines.

To be effective, each member must have confidence that other team members are capable of meeting their responsibilities. There may be concerns of legal liability for one's practice or losing control over a one to one relationship with patients. The current reimbursement structure is not designed to reward interprofessional teamwork. Time spent in team meetings is not billable. If there are not strong interprofessional working relationships among executive team members, these behaviors may not be modeled or valued.

Assessing Interprofessional Team Effectiveness

Teamwork takes practice and the ongoing support of leaders who recognize that is a huge cultural shift. Achieving a high level of interprofessional teamwork effectiveness is not without challenges. Communication breakdowns and conflict are inevitable on teams especially when members keep changing. If managed effectively, they can be viewed as an opportunity for team growth but often, this does not occur. The most common behaviors that create obstacles to effective teamwork include blaming others, turf protection, mistrust and an inability to confront issues directly. In the absence of complete trust, people are likely to withhold their ideas, observations, and questions. Professionals are also more likely to leave teams with trust issues. Trust begins with communication. Teams must be taught that relationships live within the context of conversations that teams have, or don't have with one another. When open and frank communication is not present, things can and do go wrong on teams. To evaluate the effectiveness of interprofessional teamwork, ask the following questions:[7]

1. Do team members talk about "my patient" or "our patient"?
2. Do team members clearly understand the "scope of practice" and key responsibilities of each discipline on the team?
3. Do team members know each other's names and how do they address each other?
4. Are team members respectful of other viewpoints and expertise?
5. Do team members ever round on patients together?
6. Do team members feel accountable to attend team meetings or care coordination conferences?
7. Are clear team goals established and roles assigned?
8. Can patients identify who the members of their care team are?
9. How does the team manage conflict or disagreement about care decisions?

In 2011, the Interprofessional Education Collaborative (IPEC) published the first *Core Competencies for Interprofessional Collaborative Practice*. It was updated in 2016.[8] These competencies are organized around four domains: values/ethics for interprofessional practice, roles/responsibilities, interprofessional communication, and teams and teamwork that offer a structure for best practices.[7]

- **Values/Ethics Domain Expectations** – Work with individuals of other professions to maintain a climate of mutual respect and shared values.

- **Roles/Responsibilities Domain Expectations** – Use the knowledge of one's role and those of other professions to appropriately assess and address the health care needs of patients, and to promote and advance the health of populations.

- **Interprofessional Communication Domain Expectations** – Communicate with patients, families, communities, and professionals in health and other fields in a responsive and responsible manner that supports a team approach to the promotion and maintenance of health and the prevention and treatment of disease.

- **Teams and Teamwork Expectations** – Apply relationship-building values and the principles of team dynamics to perform effectively in different team roles to plan, deliver, and evaluate patient/population-centered care and population health programs and policies that are safe, timely, efficient, effective, and equitable.

These principles are being used in academic programs today where medical students, nursing students, pharmacy, social work, and other related disciplines are taught together side by side to learn how to communicate, work in teams, and discuss pertinent issues and trends such as ethics and policy. These same principles can and should be used in any healthcare environment to build strong collaborative interprofessional teams.

REMEMBER

✓ Nurse leader coaches need to create a culture that strongly values interprofessional teamwork.

✓ A team of experts does not necessarily mean that you have an expert team.

✓ The promotion of interprofessional teamwork may involve changing current mental models about how patient care is delivered.

✓ Teamwork takes practice and the support of leaders who recognize that it is a huge cultural shift.

CHAPTER 15

AVOID TEAM DYSFUNCTION

S ometimes new leaders assume positions and find that their team has developed a culture and habits that have led to dysfunction. Assessing why teams fail and how to improve teamwork is a crucial nursing leadership skill. Will found himself in this situation when he assumed a manager position on a behavioral health unit. Given their specialty, it was somewhat surprising to him how little trust there was among team members. There were problems with communication, incivility, and lack of respect. The previous leader had a command and control style that had led to a high level of disengagement. Open and frank communication was not part of the culture. There was no sense of community and the atmosphere was negative.

Will's problems are not that unusual. Culture is described as the invisible architecture of a team or unit.[9] It is a compilation of values, behaviors, actions and group norms that ultimately become "the operating system" to use a technology metaphor. In 2002, Patrick Lencioni wrote an international business bestseller on the *Five Dysfunctions of a Team*. He notes that genuine teamwork is elusive in most organizations, yet a lack of teamwork is a primary reason why initiatives fail. He provided an overview of the following five common dysfunctions seen on teams and offered suggestions for overcoming these problems: [10]

1. AN ABSENCE OF TRUST

When team members don't trust one another, they conceal their weaknesses and mistakes. There is less willingness to ask for help or provide constructive feedback. There is a failure to tap into the expertise of others and too much time is spent on managing appearances. It is only when team members are truly comfortable with each other that they spend less time protecting themselves. Trust can be difficult to build in a dysfunctional team, but some specific suggestions include:

- Share personal histories.
- Use personality tools such as the Myers-Briggs, DISC or Strength Finders to build understanding
- Schedule experiential exercises such as a ropes course to build teamwork.
- Have each team member identify the most important contribution that each of their peers makes to the team. The team leader must be actively engaged in the process for trust to be rebuilt, and this involvement must be genuine.

2. FEAR OF CONFLICT

When there is a fear of conflict in teams, crucial conversations don't happen. Environments are created where there is a lack of transparency in how problems are managed, and personal attacks thrive. Controversial topics critical to team success are ignored. The opinions and perspectives of all team members are not considered.

To overcome a fear of conflict, team members must believe that conflict can be productive. Points of conflict need to be called out, and leaders should look for the elephants in the room. The team needs to believe that it is okay to agree to disagree. The team leader needs to practice restraint and let conflicts occur without getting prematurely involved.

3. Lack of Commitment

When teams fail to commit to a strategic direction or completion of a goal, there is ambiguity about team direction and priorities. Windows of opportunity can close because of excessive analysis or unnecessary delays. On a team that fails to commit, decisions are revisited again and again. This breeds a lack of confidence and a lack of a sense of accomplishment. Team members second guess every goal or decision. Teams need to make clear and timely decisions. Every team member needs to buy into a decision, even those who voted against it. Deadlines need to be established to reach commitment, and there needs to be recognition that there is no absolute certainty on any decision. Complete consensus will not always be possible. The team leader must be willing to push the team for closure and make decisions, even if they do turn out to be mistakes.

4. Avoidance of Accountability

When there is no accountability on teams, there is resentment among members about different standards of performance. Deadlines and key deliverables are missed. Performance measures are not achieved. There is an atmosphere of mediocrity. To avoid a lack of accountability, team members must be willing to call out their peers on behaviors that might hurt the team. Standards need to be clear, published and adhered to by all team members. The reward system should reinforce team accountability. The team leader must be willing to allow team members to hold one another accountable.

5. INATTENTION TO RESULTS

When a team is not results oriented, they will lose high performing, achievement-oriented members. Team members begin to focus on their careers and goals. The team fails to grow. When teams commit publicly to specific results, they are more likely to work passionately to achieve their goals. Reward systems should reinforce team achievement. The team leader must be willing to set a tone that focuses on results.

While these principles may sound simple, changing team behaviors can be challenging because it requires discipline and persistence. Turning around a team that is failing requires strong leadership and team commitment. However, when you consider the high costs of team failure, particularly in health care, it is a small price to pay.

CHOOSE THE RIGHT TEAM LEADER OR CHARGE NURSE

Having the right person in the right role is essential to effective teamwork. This is especially important to consider when the leadership of the team is planned. A good leader who is trusted helps the team to work in the right direction. Frontline leaders are the glue that holds units and departments together. As the span of the nurse manager role has expanded, there is increasing dependence on charge nurses and other nursing team leaders. With rising patient acuity, decreased lengths of stay, staffing shortages, pay for performance measures and new technologies, the context of healthcare environments has significantly changed, and these roles have become more complex.

When considering nurses for frontline leadership roles, research has shown that those currently working in the role rated good communication skills as a critical quality for success.[11] Communication is challenging in today's environment with both the diversity in the workforce and the culturally diverse patient populations served. Good communication is viewed as being critical to patient safety. Team leaders are expected to monitor the consistent use of communication tools that organizations have in place such as team huddles, bedside report and hourly patient rounds.

The role of the charge nurse is often described as being similar to that of an air traffic controller requiring strong organizational skills and the ability to manage their time and control their stress levels. Clinical competence in the area assigned has also been identified as being important to effectively coach and mentor others. The quality of being approachable and nonjudgmental is seen as critical. Younger, less experienced staff need to feel safe when seeking help to avoid making errors.

Once selected, team leaders need coaching. Every team leader should receive initial training in key competency areas including communication, effective teamwork, coaching and delegating, conflict management, customer service and performance management. Research findings also indicate that the ability to manage "bullying" or "horizontal violence" on teams is also a must. [11] Because we are in a rapidly changing healthcare environment, wise organizational leaders recognize that leadership development needs to be ongoing, ideally at least quarterly for team leaders. Leaders who publicly acknowledge and value the contributions of their team leaders to the success of the organization build loyalty.

DEALING WITH DYSFUNCTIONAL TEAM MEMBERS

One of the challenges for leader coaches is that you may naturally want to see the best in your staff. Karen experienced this in her role as director of a quality management department. Her team had an excellent reputation and often received praise from leaders across the medical center.

Karen knew she had one team member with a poor attitude who did not want to change, grow or work to make the team better. The achievements of the team had a "halo" effect that had protected this team member in her position.

The nurse continually failed to meet performance expectations and openly complained about her workload. Karen recognized that she could no longer avoid taking the step of removing the team member. It would be a challenging but necessary process because the nurse had been in her role for five years but a necessary one.

Failure to deal with performance problems on a team can lead strong team members to question the leader's ability. When, you have given the team member coaching and other development resources to improve and there is no change in performance, it is time to take action. Leadership expert, John Maxwell, describes this as the *law of the chain*. [1] Leaders need to recognize that the strength of the team is impacted by its weakest link.

Your Team at Night

Nursing is unusual in that much of the work is 24/7. This means that nurse leader coaches often manage teams that they may not have regular interaction with. Managers often struggle with conflicts between their day and night shift staff. You want to be supportive and visible. At the same time, you can get caught up with the chaos of the work leaving little time to think about how to best support your nurses who are managing the unit when you are not there. This can leave your night tour staff feeling isolated and disengaged. Left unchecked, you may find that you have two very different cultures on the same unit and potential differences in practice. At worst, it can lead to conflict between shifts that destroys unit morale and causes team dysfunction. The following are some dos and don'ts to consider in your leadership of night shift: [12-13]

DO

1. Keep in regular contact with the administrative supervisors who work nights to obtain their perspective on the functioning of your unit on that tour. Ask them to contact you if they see problems that you need to be aware of.
2. Schedule yourself to work all or part of the night shift quarterly. Let staff know you will be working and are there to listen to their concerns.
3. Establish some protocols for what type of situations that occur on nights that you want to be immediately notified about.
4. Demonstrate gratitude for nurses who work the night tour and recognize the inconvenience and sacrifices they make in their personal lives.
5. Monitor how staffing is done to cover night shift to ensure that staff is able to get adequate rest between tours.
6. Arrange periodic huddles with your night tour staff to communicate policy and practice changes or establish a unit Facebook® page.
7. Consider using a web platform to stream your staff meeting so your night shift can participate.
8. Maintain ongoing contact with the night charge nurses for their input into unit decisions.
9. Evaluate on an ongoing basis the workload on nights relative to admissions, discharges, transfers and workload.
10. Support your staff in their communication with physicians at night.
11. Ensure that you have night shift nurses who can serve as a strong and positive preceptor for new graduates placed on the shift.
12. Be proactive in managing any conflict that you observe between the shifts.
13. Encourage healthy habits and be an advocate for night shift in having access to cafeteria food and other amenities.

DON'T

1. Make the assumption that the workload on nights is easier.
2. Ignore signs of extreme staff fatigue or sleep deprivation and whether it is safe for a staff member to drive home.
3. Question a decision made on nights without hearing the whole story and considering the resources available.
4. Change policies or practices on the unit without input from the night tour.
5. Let practices like bedside rounding be discarded on night shift.
6. Listen to gossip from your day shift staff about what happens on nights without involving the night shift staff.
7. Place new graduates on the night shift unless there are experienced staff to coach them.
8. Lower your hiring standards because you are desperate to fill a night shift position.
9. Let conflict fester between day and night shift without intervention.
10. Destroy your personal life by responding to regular texts at night or coming in early every day to meet with night shift and then staying late.
11. Tolerate a high level of absenteeism on nights.
12. Forget to include your night shift staff in disaster and crisis training as many of these incidences occur on nights.
13. Allow night staff to opt out of self-governance initiatives.

On most 24/7 units between 30 and 40% of your staff will work the night tour. Without active collaboration with their manager, they can easily feel that they work in a different hospital than the day tour. Night shift staff play a unique role on units in keeping patients safe while the rest of the staff sleeps. They need to feel valued and respected for the work that they do.

Create a No Bullying Team Culture

Unfortunately, bullying is still prevalent in nursing teams. You may also hear this referred to as "nurses eating their young" because the victims are often new graduates. As a nurse leader, the challenge is to identify behaviors that should be characterized as bullying to stop the cycle. Nurse leaders have a responsibility to analyze the culture of units and watch carefully for verbal and non-verbal cues in the behavior of staff and on teams. Some common ones include: [14]

- Talking behind one's back instead of directly resolving conflicts.
- Making belittling comments or criticizing colleagues in front of others.
- Not sharing important information with a colleague.
- Isolating or freezing out a colleague from group activities.
- Making snide or abrupt remarks.
- Refusing to be available when a colleague needs assistance.
- Conducting acts of sabotage that deliberately set victims up for a negative situation.
- Raising eyebrows or making faces in response to the comments of colleagues.
- Failing to respect the privacy of colleagues.
- Breaking confidences.

When a team has a history of bullying, there will need to be a culture change. Part of that change is promoting a new set of shared values and goals with staff that promotes staff empowerment. communication, collaboration and life-long learning. A culture of zero-tolerance bullying is the most effective leadership strategy to prevent its occurrence. It is essential that the problem is labeled. Staff needs to be educated about the behaviors that constitute bullying to help break the silence. Raising the issue at a staff meeting and letting staff tell their stories is a crucial step to helping rebuild a culture. Staff need to know that you will quickly be responsive when you observe the behavior or when it is brought to your attention. Leaders need to engage in self-awareness activities to ensure that their own leadership style does not support bullying. The selection of preceptors who support a zero-tolerance policy is critical to orienting new staff about behavioral expectations.

When bullying is tolerated as part of the culture on a unit, it comes at a high cost to the organization, and often results in staff turnover. [14] Nurses who are victims of bullying may have problems sleeping, develop low self-esteem, exhibit depression, have poor morale and use excessive sick leave. It is also a patient safety issue when communication is compromised because of threats of bullying. Breaking the cycle on a team can help to both re-energize the staff with enthusiasm for their profession and create a healthier work environment.

REMEMBER

✓ Culture is described as the invisible architecture of a team or unit.

✓ The role of the charge nurse on a team is similar to that of an air traffic controller requiring strong organizational skills and the ability to effectively manage their time and control their stress levels.

✓ Nursing is unusual in that much of the work is 24/7. Nurse leader coaches often manage teams with whom they may not have regular interaction.

✓ Failure to deal with performance problems on a team can lead strong team members to question the leader's ability.

CHAPTER 16

RECOGNIZE EXCELLENCE

Your staff members want to be valued for their contributions to the work of the team. Leadership experts Kouzes and Posner have called this *Encouraging the Heart.* [15] *It* is one of the five exemplary practices of the world's best leaders. Leaders who encourage the heart bring others to life by recognizing their unique contributions, and who they are as individuals. Employee recognition not only recognizes the individual for his/her achievements and contributions but also serves as a critical driver of employee satisfaction, self-esteem and ongoing motivation. It is crucial to all of us that what we do matters and that our leaders will notice good work and be encouraging. Saying *thank you* may sound obvious but is often overlooked. You almost can't do it enough. A key part of encouraging the heart is to recognize contributions in a way that is valued by the person and celebrated by the team. Creating a sense of community on teams through celebrations is an important step in building commitment and social support. Leaders must be present at these events to communicate their gratitude and send a strong message about the value of the contribution. When you consider whether you as a leader do encourage the heart, ask yourself the following questions:

- Do I look for opportunities to celebrate achievements or I do I convey an attitude that the individual is just doing their job?
- Do I provide staff with specific and regular feedback about their work?
- Am I personally present when celebrations occur?
- How often do I say thank you or send a message that recognizes great performance?
- Do I look to create a spirit of community and social support in my work unit?
- How well do I know my staff?
- Do I thank staff members who have gone over and above by working overtime or changing their schedule to accommodate patient needs?
- Do I recognize preceptors for their contributions to the development of our new graduates?
- How often do I say thank you?
- Do I celebrate staff who leave my work unit for other professional development opportunities?

If you are a nurse leader working in a health system, you probably have numerous opportunities during the year to nominate your staff for awards and recognition. But do you do it? The answer for many of us is "Not as often as we should." Nurse leaders are busy. Writing a good award nomination application or letter takes time, for most nominations at least one hour. Time gets away from us and deadlines pass. Sometimes the very best nurses never get nominated for anything because no one takes the time to do it. This happened to Kaye. She had a great nurse that she wanted to nominate for her medical center's hands and heart award. This nurse not only went above and beyond for the veteran patients on her unit, but she also traveled to Puerto Rico using her own vacation time to work with victims of Hurricane Maria. The deadline for the award passed and Kaye never wrote the nomination. She was very embarrassed because she had mentioned the nomination to one of her charge nurses. The charge nurse was upset with her failure to follow through.

Some guidelines with recognition feedback include the following:

- Don't delay praise, do it sooner rather than later.
- Do it because you are appreciative and be sincere.
- Be as specific as possible by providing details of what has led to the recognition.
- Make it personal, either in person or a hand-written note.
- Don't mix criticism and praise.

INVEST IN WRITING AWARD NOMINATIONS

It is essential that we begin to think of awards as an investment because even a nomination can be significantly meaningful to a nurse or other staff member. Researchers, Kelly, Runge and Spencer looked at the predictors of compassion fatigue and compassion satisfaction in acute care nurses. [16] In their work, they found that meaningful recognition (which in this study was identified as a nomination for the Daisy Award) had a significant impact on reducing burnout, increasing satisfaction, and improving retention, especially in the Millennial nurse cohort. But knowing that these awards make a difference does not make them easier to write. Some leaders may write the nominations without telling the employee that they are doing it. While surprise awards are great, asking the nurse for input can make the application much richer. For major awards, you should ask nurses for their updated resumes and one or two stories about the outcomes of their contributions. Putting a great nomination together with this information becomes much easier. Some additional tips include:

- Create a timeline and start early so you don't miss the deadline.
- Make sure the nurse meets all the criteria for the award.
- Include outcomes and contributions that relate directly to each of the criteria outlined for the award.
- Include stories and use examples to illustrate key points and demonstrate the passion of the applicant.
- Fill out every section in the award application – they are generally individually scored.
- Choose your words carefully as words have power – Use words that are powerful such as "a can-do attitude" – "strong ability to connect with patients and families" – "unselfishly gives his/her time or energy" – "ignites engagement of others" – "committed professional" – "transformational leader" or a "generous mentor" Accompany them with specific examples of behaviors to illustrate how.
- Write in an active voice and use the nurse's name frequently throughout the narrative.
- Pay attention to word count because if you go beyond the word count, everything may not appear in the final application.
- Proof-read everything you write.
- See every award as an opportunity to nominate one of your staff.

The next time you receive an award announcement that one or more of your staff would qualify for, don't bypass the email or put the flyer under a stack of papers. See it as an investment opportunity to make your team stronger. Take the time to decide who your best candidates are, ask for their input and write the nomination. You won't be sorry you did.

INDIVIDUALIZE RECOGNITION

In their book *How Full is Your Bucket,* authors Tom Rath and Donald Clifton recommend flipping the golden rule when it comes to recognition. [17] So instead of doing unto others as you would have them do unto you, do unto others as they would have you do unto them. Individualization is the key when it comes to rewards and recognition. It is powerful when leaders provide recognition in a way that is meaningful to their employees. Some of your staff will want tangible awards or gifts. For others, a note of thanks or words of recognition will matter most. Even the forum in which recognition is given should be considered. Some staff members love public recognition of their achievements while others would prefer to get it in a one to one conversation.

It is impossible to provide individualized recognition without asking staff questions about their preferences. Here's a set of questions you can ask each of your direct reports, one-on-one:

- What contributions/successes do you want to be recognized for?
- When you accomplish something worthy of recognition, whom do you want to know it?
- What's the best gesture of recognition you've ever received? Why was it the best?
- What form of recognition is most meaningful to you?

SHINE A LIGHT – DON'T CAST A SHADOW

Leaders sometimes think that they will lose power if they are not on center stage to accept the accolades for team success when quite the opposite is true. They may also feel a sense of entitlement in owning all of the team's achievements. When leaders behave this way, it erodes trust on the team. A lack of trust has a serious impact on staff morale and engagement. Poor morale can lead to more mistakes, less productivity, and increased employee turnover. Besides if not heeded, minor grumblings from staff members can spiral into dissension and more significant problems.

All staff wants to be valued for their contributions to the work of the team. When leaders fail to say thank you or take the recognition for themselves, staff feel devalued. The inability to give others the credit and praise that they deserve is a serious leadership career derailer. True leadership influence is built by making others successful. It is about seeking opportunities to create mutual benefit and building and nurturing relationships. Marshall Goldsmith, a nationally recognized leadership coach, observes that successful people become great leaders when they shift the focus from themselves to others.[18] Some important ways to shine the light on your staff for team accomplishments include:

1. Have staff present to accept awards when given for team accomplishments.
2. Have staff present the outcomes of successful initiatives to senior management.
3. Have staff present with you at professional conferences where you discuss unit or department initiatives.
4. Make staff recognition a part of every staff meeting.
5. Introduce high performing staff to others as "a superstar."
6. Let staff know you see the potential they have and that you want to develop it.
7. Take time out to recognize staff achievements such as certification or advanced education.

Smart managers learn quickly that one of the most significant forms of employee acknowledgment and recognition occurs when a manager gives credit publicly where credit is due. The essence of leadership is to get work done through the efforts of others. If you are a leader who casts a shadow rather than shines a light, it is never too late to change your behavior. The rewards will be a more positive work culture with better outcomes. You will also be seen as a more authentic leader.

Remember

✓ Encouraging the heart through recognition is one of the five exemplary practices of the world's best leaders.

✓ It is important that we begin to think of awards as an investment because even a nomination can be significantly meaningful to a nurse or other staff member.

✓ It is powerful when leaders provide recognition in a way that is meaningful to their employees.

✓ Smart managers learn quickly that one of the most significant forms of employee acknowledgment and recognition occurs when a manager gives credit publicly where credit is due.

CHAPTER 17

Build Individual and Team Resilience

With the uncertainty in healthcare and concern about the financial health of organizations, it is not surprising that both nurses and their leaders feel stressed and burned out. Dr. Donald Berwick, the former CEO of the Institute for Healthcare Improvement (IHI), observed that it seems paradoxical in healthcare where caring should be the focus that so many healthcare professionals are experiencing burnout and a loss of joy in their work. [19] In the whitepaper, *The IHI Framework for Improving Joy in Work*, the authors noted that if burnout in healthcare was described in clinical or public health terms, it might well be called an epidemic. [20] Building individual and team resiliency has never been more important. Nurse leader coaches play a crucial role in helping staff to adapt to changes in their environments and develop a resiliency muscle.

Resiliency helps us to bounce back from stressors and serious challenges in our lives. You have probably seen examples with your staff of situations where individuals suffer enormous setbacks yet are somehow able to recover from their problems and even emerge stronger. Personal resiliency is deeply rooted in the habits of our mind as much as our values and beliefs. It is shaped by our personal experiences with adversity, our natural levels of optimism, the level of impact that an experience has on our lives, our social support system and our propensity to ruminate.[21] Being attentive to building your resiliency has never been more important especially for our younger nursing workforce. The American Psychological Association reports that 12% of Millennials have been diagnosed with an anxiety disorder, which is considerably higher than older generations.[22]

If we want our staff to have long and productive careers, it is vital to help them to develop resiliency. As a leader coach, you will never be able to eliminate all of the stresses and challenges in the work environment. When staff members are more resilient, they have the strength to tackle their problems head-on and manage adversity with less stress. The good news is that resiliency is like a muscle. It grows as we learn to successfully navigate negative situations. How we view adversity and stress strongly impacts our capacity to bounce back. Martin Seligman, a psychiatrist and national expert on resilience, believes that reframing how we explain setbacks to ourselves is the key to developing resilience.[23] Situations are rarely as good or bad as we may describe them. When you are resilient, you recognize that both positive and negative experiences can lead to transformational growth.

Coaching to Reflect on Challenging Situations

To help staff gain clarity on stressful situations, you can use the same three-step coaching framework developed by the Center for Creative

Leadership that we discussed in Chapter 2. Your questions could include the following: [24]

Describe for me what happened to you.

Ask the staff member to tell you the story of what happened as objectively as possible sticking to the facts. Include key details such as who was involved, where did it happen and when did it happen.

Tell me about your reaction to what happened.

Ask the staff member to describe their reaction to the event or experience as factually and objectively as possible. How did they respond? What were their thoughts and emotional feelings?

What were your lessons learned in this situation?

Ask the staff member what they learned from both the situation and their reaction to it. Have they identified some development needs that they might have to better cope with such events in the future? Is there a pattern in the way they reacted to events? What would they do differently in the situation occurred again?

Jackie put this coaching guidance to work in a situation with one of her new graduate nurses. The young nurse took every corrective criticism personally and had become very anxious and fearful about career failure. Jackie talked with her to understand her self-limiting beliefs about criticism. She equated corrective feedback with failure as a professional. This was catastrophic thinking. She spent too much time ruminating about events at work. Rumination is taking a stressful event in your life and churning it over and over in your mind with *what if* or *if only* questions. This rumination leads to higher levels of stress and makes it challenging to be resilient. Jackie worked with her to help her quiet her mind and be present to help her break the cycle of rumination. They also talked about lessons learned in every situation and how they could be applied in the future.

THE RESILIENCY TOOLBOX

There are evidence-based strategies that can help you and your staff to become more resilient. These include the following: [21]

HAVE AN ATTITUDE OF GRATITUDE.

There is strong evidence that gratitude promotes adaptive coping and personal growth. Being grateful makes us resilient by keeping us hopeful. It reminds us that we have the power to act and expands our possibilities. A widely used gratitude technique is listing three things daily that you are grateful for in your life or that have gone well in your day. Some nursing units and departments have made this part of their end of shift huddle. This is a positive way to end the workday.

FOCUS ON YOUR STRENGTHS AND PAST SUCCESSES.

Drawing on your past successes can help to restore your self-confidence. There is also strong evidence that knowing your strengths and talents and putting them to work can help to power you through challenging situations.

PRACTICE MEDITATION OR YOGA.

When your self-confidence is challenged, you can quickly shift to worse-case scenarios by ruminating about the past or worrying about the future. Yoga and meditation are both designed to shift our attention to the present moment and reduce our anxiety about the what-ifs. These practices force us to relax and slow down time by being in the moment.

ADOPT GOOD PERSONAL WELLNESS HABITS.

There are strong correlations between resiliency and our wellness habits. Sleeping seven hours each night, eating a balanced diet, seeking fun in your life and exercising all promote higher levels of resiliency. Taking time to do self-care is especially important during challenging times to reduce our stress levels.

Develop a strong social support system.

It can be very challenging to rebuild your self-confidence without someone to be your cheerleader and accountability partner. Although you may find it difficult to confide your struggles to others especially if you are known for your self-confidence, it is essential to reach out to family, friends and professional colleagues. Connecting with others can keep us from wallowing in our situation. Sharing our goals moving forward with a trusted friend can help us to get back on track.

Social Capital on Teams Creates Higher Resiliency

In a popular TED talk titled, *Forget the pecking order at work*, Margaret Hefferman a business thought leader talks about the importance of building social capital on teams as a way to promote resiliency during challenging times.[25] Social capital is defined as the reliance and interdependency that happens on teams when trust is built. It is social capital that allows teams to work through conflict, survive turbulent times and ultimately achieve more collectively. Teams with more social capital have higher resiliency. It takes a leader who values the importance of social capital to strategically help teams to build it through the construction of stronger social networks. Nurse leader coaches can help their teams to build social capital by doing the following:

1. **Create Opportunities for Staff to Better Know One Another.**

   Repeat exposure to others can help to build trust. It might surprise you how little nursing team members know about one another in some environments. Nurse leaders can help build community by creating opportunities for staff to learn more about one another and what is important to them in their work. Huddles and staff meetings can be great opportunities to have staff tell something about themselves, what is important to them and share their uniqueness. Leaders should also take the time themselves to learn about the lives of their staff, the names of their children and special days such as birthdays. In today's environment, many staff live alone and may not have close family or friends. For these staff, work is an important connection.

2. Promote Inclusiveness on the Team.

To build strong teams, everyone must feel like a valued member. Resilient teams have fewer superstars and more team players. Inclusiveness means acknowledging everyone who contributes to the team including interdisciplinary team members, housekeeping and engineering.

3. Encourage an Environment of Trust.

Social capital is built in an environment of trust. Conflict on teams is natural and should not be discouraged but it is important that it is managed respectfully. Nurse leaders can help foster this trust by refusing to engage in gossip, speculation or criticism of others. Leaders set the tone for the culture by insisting that all parties are present for the discussion and no conclusions are drawn until the full story is heard.

4. Look for Opportunities to Celebrate and Gather as a Community

Celebrating special events, birthdays and staff achievements is an important part of establishing a sense of community. Most nurse leaders would readily agree that the importance of sharing meals cannot be underestimated in establishing staff camaraderie. Participation in community events such as heart walks or other fund raising drives can be a great way to build team camaraderie and social capital.

There is strong evidence that teams with strong social capital are more resilient. They also outperform those teams with less. Historically, the way teams have been managed in organizations pits staff against one another. Reducing rivalry and replacing it with social capital has the potential to result in better outcomes. By making your workplace and team membership more enjoyable, you may be able to boost employee morale and improve your staff satisfaction. A sense of team togetherness is energizing to staff, reduces absenteeism and improves patient care.

RESPONDING TO MORAL DISTRESS ON TEAMS

Sometimes work stress is directly related to moral distress that healthcare team members may experience in caring for patients. Maria has this issue on her medical-surgical unit. Her patient population includes a high case mix of elderly patients covered by Medicare. Many of these patients are close to the end of life, yet are undergoing invasive and sometimes futile treatment. They often don't have families geographically close who can advocate for them. Nurses find themselves involved in giving treatments that will have little impact on the patient's outcome, and may even lead to a more uncomfortable death. Sometimes they have strong feelings about what ethical action is appropriate in the situation, but are unable to act on it. This results in moral distress. Situations like Maria's staff is experiencing are serious dilemmas faced each day by practicing nurses. Unlike problems which are more easily solvable, dilemmas are challenging situations with differing points of view, and often no perfect answer.

Nurses feel moral distress when they have strong feelings about the ethically appropriate action in a situation but are unable to act on it. They proceed to give care that is contrary to their personal and professional values. This undermines the nurse's sense of integrity and authenticity. There are sources of moral distress other than end of life challenges. Conflict with physicians, bullying in the workplace, challenges to religious beliefs and system decisions that negatively impact care can all cause moral distress. Responses to moral distress can be physical, emotional, behavioral or spiritual. Evidence-based studies have established a relationship between the level of moral distress and intent to stay in a practice setting or even the profession itself.

Moral distress can cause the following problems in the work environment:

- Team stress
- Poor communication
- Lack of trust
- Defensiveness
- Lack of collaboration
- High turnover rates

THE 4 A's MODEL

Although moral distress can occur in any setting, critical care units are ground zero. This is because of the sheer number of end-of-life and aggressive treatment decisions that must be made daily on critically ill patients. Not surprisingly, the American Association of Critical Care developed a framework called the 4 A Model. The purpose of the model is to help nurses and leaders assess and take action when situations causing moral distress occur in the workplace. [26]

Ask – Nurse leaders should observe for signs on moral distress on their teams and if unsure ask. The goal is to identify when it is present.

Affirm – After validating the feelings of staff that they are feeling moral distress, commit to address the concerns and affirm the professional obligation to act ethically.

Assess – Assess the extent of the problem causing staff moral distress. What are the risks and benefits of taking action to reduce moral stress. Assess whether there is a leadership imperative to move to the next stage which is the action stage.

Act – This is the stage where the leader would begin to initiate change that is needed to reduce moral distress. There may be a need for the ethics committee to become involved in end-of-life care or perhaps there is a better way to involve families in decision making. It might include an educational program for staff or a quality improvement project.

Addressing moral distress requires making changes. Nurse leaders are in an excellent position to provide a sounding board for staff on helping them to manage these dilemmas. By helping to alleviate or lesson moral distress that staff feels, you can improve nurse resiliency, and retention, and ultimately improve care.

PROMOTE CARING FOR SELF

Self-care is crucial to staying resilient in one's work. Nurse leaders need to role model self-care behaviors for staff. Kim Richards owns the Self-Care Academy and coaches nurses and leaders on self-care. [27] In her work, she uses a six-part framework to self-care developed by Barbara Dossey, an expert in holistic nursing. [28] The pathways include physical care of self, maintaining mental health, cultivating emotional awareness, attending to one's spiritual needs, building and maintaining close personal relationships and recognizing the power of choice. Richards cites important reasons to invest in self-care especially in today's chaotic healthcare environment.

1. **Rest is an investment in yourself,
   your team and your future.**
   We know from work studies involving nurses that a lack of rest
   leads to fatigue, problems with concentration, difficulty controlling
   emotions and poor decision making. Leaders experience these problems too when they work long hours and stimulate themselves with
   caffeine to keep going. Caring for self is not selfish behavior on the
   part of leaders. This investment in rest will make you feel better,
   be more alert and better able to process the many challenges that
   leaders confront today.

2. **Recharging your battery will
   make you a better leader.**
   Leaders sometimes worry about what will happen if they take time
   off. The reality is that recharging your battery will both make you
   a better leader and reduce the likelihood of role burnout. Taking
   periodic planned vacations is very important. This recharging of your
   mind, body and emotions allows you to be at your best so you can
   be of service to others. Over the course of their careers, nurse leaders
   learn that life and work move on even in their absence. Wise leaders
   know that often the most reliable gauge of their leadership is how
   well they have developed others to function when they are not there.

3. **Find an activity outside of work
   that brings you self-renewal.**
   As a leader, you should take the time to find at least one activity outside of work that quiets your mind, soothes your soul and
   re-energizes you. This activity could be meditation, yoga, walking,
   reading, cooking or prayer. The choice of activity is personal, but it
   should be something that enhances your well-being and something
   you can commit to frequently doing.

4. **Make time to reflect on how you use your time and energy at work.**

During a 2005 commencement address, Steve Jobs the former CEO of Apple spoke about how remembering that he would soon be dead is the most important tool that he had encountered to help him make the big choices in life. He told these graduating students that *"all external expectations, all pride, all fear of embarrassment or failure – these things just fall away in the face of death, leaving only what is truly important. Remembering that you are going to die is the best way I know to avoid the trap of thinking that you have something to lose. You are already naked. There is no reason not to follow your heart".*[29] This is good advice for nurse leaders who sometimes believe that their units or departments cannot function without them or are hesitant to change their work patterns. Time in self-reflection is an essential step in learning how to re-balance your work and life.

5. **Leaders set the example for self-care on their teams.**

If it appears to your staff that self-care and leadership are mutually exclusive from observing your behaviors, then this will be the impression that they have about leadership. To achieve a healthy work environment, leaders need to promote the idea of self-care and role modeling is a powerful way to do this. Attention to our self-care will both keep us resilient and establish it as a strong value in our work culture.

Remember

✓ Nurse leader coaches play a key role in helping staff to adapt to changes in their environments and build a resiliency muscle.

✓ Resiliency is like a muscle, it grows as we learn to successfully navigate negative situations.

✓ It is social capital that allows teams to work through conflict, survive turbulent times and ultimately achieve more collectively.

✓ Sometimes work stress is directly related to moral distress that healthcare team members may experience in caring for patients.

CHAPTER 18

LET TEAM MEMBERS GROW AND SOMETIMES GO

This is our final chapter. The focus in this last section of the book is how nurse leader coaches can help staff to grow in their careers. Leaders are sometimes reluctant to do this because there are risks that staff might leave the unit or organization. In some cases, this may happen. However, we also know that the frontline leader is the linchpins in staff retention. Part of what will build loyalty is a strong interest in developing the skills of your staff. As a leader coach, you must recognize that if you focus on the personal, professional and career development of your team, they will feel cared for and this will translate to better care for patients. This sometimes means that you may lose some of your best staff, but it is a risk worth taking.

This is the situation that Marla confronted in her role as a critical care director. She overheard Jake, one of her strongest nurses, talking with a professional colleague about his interest in artificial intelligence

(AI) and robotics. He mentioned to his colleague that he had a career goal to eventually work at the intersection of healthcare and AI. He was reading everything he could on the topic but was unsure about his next steps. Marla had a choice to make at that point. No one would have faulted her if she ignored the conversation. However, she chose not to do that. She dreaded the possibility that she could lose such a valuable employee but Marla also cared about Jake as a person. As a leader coach, she wanted to see him achieve his professional goals. Marla chose the route of career coaching because that is what Jake needed. She talked with the director of technology in her health system, and he agreed to mentor Jake to develop in his interest area. Jake was excited, engaged and appreciated Marla's efforts. He shared his career development plan with others on the staff. While it is true that he will probably leave the unit to achieve career growth, he may not have to leave the organization. Marla will have played a key role in his future professional legacy.

Career Coaching

Marla recognized that having career coaching conversations with her staff would achieve several goals. They can help you as the leader better understand career values, motivators and even the skills that they would like to develop while working on your unit. There is enormous power in these discussions because it conveys to your staff that you have a personal interest in supporting their development. Not all staff will be equally interested in career coaching. Nurses look for different things at different points in their careers. Some will want to grow their careers while others may want to slow down or even cut back on responsibilities at work. Before leaders can initiate career coaching, you need a good sense of the staff member's goals, interests, and values. You also need to consider what developmental activities are available in the work environment. Examples of developmental activities include:

- Emerging leader development courses
- Specialty training
- A mentorship program
- Support for certification
- Participation on task forces and committees
- Stretch assignments

Leaders can use the GROW framework that we talked about earlier in the book to explore career development. Figure 18-1 illustrates some good exploratory coaching questions. [30]

PROMOTE NETWORKING

Building a strong professional network is critical to professional success yet few leaders encourage or teach their staff how to do this. It is surprising how many nurses have few contacts outside their healthcare organization. Many nurses never make the investment of getting involved with professional associations or take the time to ensure that they have a strong network of colleagues both within and outside their organization. They wonder why they should spend their free time on an activity that seems so indirectly related to the work that they do. They fail to see how a network can not only enhance their professional growth but also prove to be a wise career investment. When they hit a roadblock in their career, they may be shut off from their professional colleagues, and not have anyone to seek guidance from about their next steps.

Today's healthcare environments are volatile and building a strong network can serve as an insurance policy. Harvey McKay, a master networker, has advised that you dig your well before you are thirsty. [31] This is good advice in today's environment where so many jobs are never advertised and recruiters rely heavily on referrals from professionals they trust. A nurse that is interested in developing specific skills or advancing

FIGURE 18-1
GROW MODEL CAREER
COACHING QUESTIONS

G *Goal*	• What is your overall goal for your career? • What would like to be doing five years from now? • How will you know when you have achieved your career goals? • What is the most important thing in your nursing practice? • How do you think your current role can contribute to your career goals?
R *Reality*	• What do you love about your current position? • What would you like to change about your current role? • Are there skills that you would like to develop that you don't already have? • Is there anything you need to change to get where you would like to go with your career? • What is getting in the way of your career goals so far?
O *Options*	• What roles in nursing would you like to learn more about? • What ideas do you have to further develop your knowledge, skills, and abilities? • What can we do within the context of your current role to help you on your career journey?
W *Way Forward*	• How much of your own time and resources are you willing to commit to your career growth? • What can you do next to help you move forward with your career goals? • What might get in the way of your achieving your goals? How can you overcome that? • What are you going to do next of the things we have talked about? • What support do you need from me to move forward?

her education can utilize her professional network to identify a mentor for skill development or guidance on educational opportunities.

Nurse leader coaches can encourage membership in professional associations as an excellent way to begin networking. Attendance at conferences provides an ideal place to start to build a network. Networking is an active behavior designed to build relationships. Nurse leaders can coach staff in how to do this by helping staff see the opportunities to jump-start careers by becoming involved in committees in organizations, participating in projects and running for office. When staff attends conferences, they should be encouraged to set goals to meet and talk with at least three new people each day. Even if you are introverted and hate the prospect of networking, you can never go wrong asking questions. People love to talk about themselves. Some good questions to get the conversation started could include:[32]

- How did you get started in your role?
- What are your challenges?
- What significant changes do you see in your environment?
- What is the most innovative thing that is happening in your organization?
- What do you think will happen with healthcare reform?
- What trends do you see happening in nursing today?
- What advice would you give to an emerging nurse leader?
- How can I help you?
- Who else do you know at this meeting that would be helpful for me to talk with?

Professional preparation for networking also includes making sure that you are professionally attired and have business cards to share contact information. Networking is a learned skill and nurse leaders who coach staff on how to more effectively network will help them to build career success.

Pushing Staff out of the Nest

Sometimes leaders need to push their staff out of the nest to promote their career development. Vickie found herself in this position. One of her staff, Carole, had asked to attend the emerging leader course in her health system. Carole did well in the program and was identified as a high potential future leader in her organization. Six months after taking the class, she still has not applied for any leadership openings. Vickie set up a coaching session with Carole to find out what was holding her back. She learned that Carole feared the loss of her comfort zone. She had worked on the unit for five years and was worried about leaving behind valued colleagues and well-established routines. Carole's rationale was congruent with what we learned earlier in the book about our work lives as a series of habits, both good and bad that we develop over time.

Habits are the brain's way of saving energy. Whenever we try to change something in our lives (such as Carole leaving her unit to take a leadership role), it means changing habits. This can only happen with very intentional work because new habits require extensive practice. [33] The prospect of doing something new or different can be stressful. Many of us have a bias to maintain the status quo because it is easier. When we consider whether or not to move to another position, we often think about what we are leaving behind. This is where Vickie began with her coaching of Carole. They discussed the significant contributions that she had made to the unit but then shifted to what she wanted for the future.

Vickie asked Carole some great reflective questions including:

- What is on your mind about your career?
- What do you want to be different in the next 3-5 years of your career?
- What are your fears about taking a leadership role?
- How could you make a difference as a leader?
- How can I help you on your path forward?

Staying in a situation also means that you are potentially giving up some great opportunities to contribute and be more productive if you did make a change. Carole could find that leaving her current unit would open exciting new possibilities and lead to incredible growth opportunities. She will never know this if she does not pursue other position options. Sometimes it is the leader coach who needs to push staff out of the nest.

MANAGING RESIGNATIONS WITH GRACE

Many managers dread when staff walk into their office and say, *I need to talk with you about something*. They fear that *something* will be a resignation and sometimes it is. In today's workplace with nurse vacancy rates hovering around 10%, losing an experienced staff member can present significant staffing challenges. Even with these challenges, resignations should be managed with intention. A wise mentor once told me that a resignation should be viewed in some ways like a funeral. She observed that *"How you behave – is a tribute not only to the person leaving but to everyone left behind."* I have always found this to be good advice. Once a staff member has decided to resign regardless of how inconvenient it is for you as the manager, how you behave says a great deal about you as a leader. It impacts how honest employees will be with you if they are considering other career opportunities and whether you are seen as someone who supports professional growth. Staff may choose to resign for many reasons, some of which you will have no control over. Leaders who feel that a resignation indicates disloyalty acquire a reputation as angry and vindictive.

Managing resignations with grace is an important leadership behavior. Your leadership behaviors should include the following:

• Acknowledge their contributions and how they will be missed.

- Ask if there is anything you can do to change their mind (If you want to).
- Work with them on a transition date and any benefits they may be entitled to.
- Keep the lines of communication completely open.

Your staff will carefully watch how you respond when someone leaves. Do you demonstrate grace and gratitude or do you behave in a way that seems angry and reactive? Ultimately for the good of your unit or department, you want your staff member feeling good about the workplace and ready to recommend it to others that might be interested. If you stay in your leadership role long enough, you may even be surprised at how many staff often return to their former positions when they find out the grass is not greener somewhere else.

Many employers now have very active strategies to stay in contact with staff who have left and invite them back. Nurse leaders who don't already do this should strongly consider the five following ways that they can leave the door open for staff to return:

1. Before the staff member leaves, sit down with them and wish them the very best. End the conversation by saying that "Sometimes new positions don't work out as well as we think they will and if this happens, please call me." Don't ever bad mouth the new employer.
2. Leave a great last impression by giving them a going away party and thanking them for their contributions.
3. Ask to connect with the staff member on LinkedIn – this will give you access so you can see how they are progressing in their career and send congratulatory messages.
4. Don't hold grudges against staff who leave and speak highly of them to their co-workers who probably do stay in touch with them.

5. Send holiday messages and if the staff member has had a major tragic life event – reach out.

How you manage staff who leave speaks volumes about your leadership. If you lose a staff member, keep in mind that it does not have to be forever. Great supportive leader coaches are unfortunately in short supply but staff often don't realize this until they leave so keep the door open.

REMEMBER

✓ There is enormous power in these career coaching conversations because it conveys to your staff that you have a personal interest in supporting their development.

✓ Sometimes leaders need to push their staff out of the nest to promote their career development.

✓ Building a strong professional network is critical to professional success yet few leaders encourage or teach their staff how to do this.

✓ How you manage staff after they resign speaks volumes about your leadership.

FINAL THOUGHTS

Now it's your turn. Becoming a nurse leader coach requires a change in your leadership behavior. Any new change in behavior can be challenging until it becomes routine so you will need to practice the skills presented in this book. Start with small changes. Choose two things you will do differently in your leadership. Zig Ziglar, a great motivation expert, once said that *"you don't have to be great to get started but you do have to get started to be great."* If you commit yourself to become a nurse leader coach, you will become the boss that no one wants to leave. So, get started on your journey. It will make you a better nurse leader and a better person.

REFERENCES – PART 3

1. Maxwell J. *The 17 Indisputable Laws of Teamwork: Embrace Them and Empower Your Team.* New York: Harper Collins; 2013.
2. Grubaugh ML, Flynn L. Relationships among nurse manager leadership skills, conflict management and unit teamwork. *Journal of Nursing Administration.* 48(7), 383-388; 2018.
3. Society Human Resource Management. *Developing and Sustaining High Performance Work Teams.* Available at https://www.shrm.org/resourcesandtools/tools-and-samples/toolkits/pages/developingandsustaininghigh-performanceworkteams.aspx Accessed September 22nd, 2018.
4. Zemke R, Raines C, Filipczak, B. *Generations at Work: Managing the Clash of Veterans, Boomers, Xers and Nexters in Your Workplace.* Amacon Publishers; 1999.
5. Meister JC, Willyerd K. *The 2020 Workplace: How Innovative Companies Attract, Develop and Keep Tomorrow's Employees Today.* New York: Harper Business; 2010.
6. Janis, I. L. Groupthink. *Psychology Today.* 5(6): 43–46, 74–76; 1971.

7. *Interprofessional Education Collaborative Expert Panel. (2011). Core competencies for interprofessional collaborative practice: Report of an expert panel. Washington, D.C.: Interprofessional Education Collaborative.* Available at https://www.aacom.org/docs/default-source/insideome/ ccrpt05-10-11.pdf?sfvrsn=77937f97_2

8. *Interprofessional Education Collaborative. (2016). Core Competencies for Interprofessional Collaborative Practice Washington, D.C.: Interprofessional Education Collaborative.* Available https://nebula. wsimg.com/2f68a39520b03336b41038c370497473?AccessKeyId= DC06780E69ED19E2B3A5&disposition=0&alloworigin=1

9. Tye J, Dent B. Building a Culture of Ownership in Healthcare: The Invisible Architecture of Core Values, Attitude and Self-Empowerment. Indianapolis: Sigma Theta Tau; 2017.

10. Lencoioni P. *The Five Dysfunctions of a Team.* San Francisco: Jossey-Bass Publishers; 2002.

11. Schwarzkopf R., Sherman, R O, Kiger, A. Taking charge: Frontline nurse leader development. *Journal of the Continuing Education in Nursing, 43*(4),154-160; 2012.

12. Claffey C. Nursing in the dark: Leadership support for night shift. *Nursing Management. 37*(5); 41-44; 2006.

13. Weaver S, Lindgren T G, Cadmus E, Flynn F, Thomas-Hawkins C. Report from the night shift: How administrative supervisors achieve nurse and patient safety. *Nursing Administration Quarterly. 41*(4); 328-36; 2017.

14. Longo J, Sherman R O. Leveling horizontal violence. *Nursing Management, 38*(3), 34-37; 50-51; 2007.

15. Kouzes JM, Posner BZ. *The Leadership Challenge 6ᵗʰ Edition.* Hoboken NJ: John Wiley & Sons; 2017.

16. Kelly L, Runge J, Spencer C. Predictors of compassion fatigue and compassion satisfaction in Acute Care Nurses. *Journal of Nursing Scholarship, 47*(6), 522-28; 2015.

17. Rath T, Clifton DO. *How Full is Your Bucket: Positive Strategies for Work and Life.* New York: Gallup Press; 2004.

18. Goldsmith M. *What Got You Here Won't Get You There.* New York: Hyperion; 2007.

19. Berwick, D.M. (2017). *Forward.* As cited in Perlo, J., et al. *IHI Framework for Improving Joy in Work.* IHI White Paper. Cambridge, MA: Institute for Healthcare Improvement.

20. Perlo, J., Balik, B., Swenson, S., Kabcenell, A., Landsman, J. & Feeley, D. (2017). *IHI*

21. *Framework for Improving Joy in Work.* IHI White Paper. Cambridge, MA: Institute for

22. Healthcare Improvement. Available at www.ihi.org.

23. Sherman RO. Building your resiliency. *American Nurse Today, 13*(9), 26-28; 2018.

24. American Psychological Association . *Stress by Generation.* 2012 Available at http://www.apa.org/news/press/releases/stress/2012/generations.aspx

25. Seligman MEP. *The hope circuit: A psychologist's journey from helplessness to optimism.* New York: Hatchett; 2018.

26. Roger D, Petrie N. *Work with stress: Building a resilient mindset for lasting success.* New York: McGraw-Hill; 2017.

27. Hefferman M. (June 16, 2015 Ted Talk). *Forget the pecking order at work* Available at https://www.ted.com/talks/margaret_heffernan_why_it_s_time_to_forget_the_pecking_order_at_work

28. McCue C. Using the AACN framework to alleviate moral distress. *Online Journal of Issues in Nursing. 16*(1); 2010. Available at http://ojin.nursingworld.org/MainMenuCategories/EthicsStandards/Resources/Courage-and-Distress/AACN-Framework-and-Moral-Distress.html

29. Richards, K. (2012). To care for others, we must FIRST care for ourselves. *Reflections on Nursing Available at https://www.reflectionson nursingleadership.org/features/more-features/Vol38-2-nurses-to-care-for-others-we-must-first-care-for-ourselves-(part-two)*

30. Dossey BM, Keegan L. *Holistic nursing: A handbook for practice* (6th ed.). Burlington, MA: Jones & Bartlett Learning; 2013.

31. Jobs S. (Stanford Commencement 2005). https://www.bing.com/videos/search?q=steve+jobs+2005+stanford+commencement+speech&view=detail&mid=256ECF6D1209B7AF39EF256ECF6D1209B7AF39EF&FORM=VIRE

32. Jackson K. *Essential Questions to Grow Your Team.* Careerbalance LTD; 217.

33. Mackay H. *Dig your well before you are thirsty: The only networking book you'll ever need.* New York: Currency Press; 1999.

34. Sherman RO, Cohen TM. Why your nursing networks matter. *American Nurse Today, 13*(3), 9-11; 2018.

35. Duhigg, C. *The Power of Habit: Why We do What We do in Life and Business.* New York: Random House; 2012.

PART 4

THE COACHING TOOLBOX

"What we know matters but who
we are matters more."

BRENE BROWN

GROW MODEL COACHING TEMPLATE

Name: _____   Date: _____

GROW Model Step	Questions to Ask	Coach Notes Column
GOAL **Type Clarification** • Professional Goal • Personal Well-Being • Performance Goal • Long-Term Goal • Session Goal	• What would you like to talk about? • What do you hope to achieve, resolve or solve? • What do you want to accomplish in this session? • Why is this goal important to you now? • What would you like to happen that is not happening now? • How will we know if we have met your goal expectations?	
REALITY • Clarify current situation • Check assumptions • Identify Obstacles (time, money, environment, people, self-beliefs)	• What is happening now? • What is getting in the way of your goals? • How do you know this is accurate? • What impact or effect does this have? • What have you tried so far? • What personal changes will you need to make?	

GROW Model Step	Questions to Ask	Coach Notes Column
OPTIONS • Brainstorm Choices • Select Preferred Options	• What approaches could you use? • What have you done in similar situations? • What is your preferred option? • Who might be able to help you? • What is your preferred option? • What will happen if you do nothing?	
WAY FORWARD • An Action Plan • Commitment to Action • Time Sensitive Actions • Clear Outcomes	• What is your first step? • What is your timeframe? • What could get in the way? • How will you know you are successful? • What support do you need? • What follow-up should we plan?	

Coaching Guide Nurse Leader Coach ™

POWERFUL COACHING QUESTIONS

PROFESSIONAL GROWTH QUESTIONS

What gets you excited about the work you do?

What are your strengths?

What one professional goal do you have for the next six months?

What steps have you taken to achieve your goal?

What is the real challenge here for you?

What is on your mind?

How can I help you?

What can I do as a manager to bring out your personal best?

What would you like me to know about you that I don't know?

What can you contribute to the unit?

PERFORMANCE MANAGEMENT QUESTIONS

Tell me what happened here?

What don't I know about this situation?

What impact did your behavior have on others in this situation?

How do you know that your perceptions are accurate?

What could you have done differently in this situation?

What have you learned from what happened here?

How would you handle this situation in the future?

How can we fix this?

What events or choices led you to this place?

What do you need from me to help you be successful?

What is the best recognition that you have ever received?

How can you use your strengths in this situation?

Career Development Questions

What do you want in your career?

What career goals have you established for yourself?

What have you done to learn more about these career goals?

What support do you need to achieve your goals?

What obstacles do you see in achieving this goal?

Who could help you in your career planning?

What is your first step to put your goals into action?

How will that action help meet your goal?

What have you already tried to achieve your goals?

How can we make this goal measurable?

How will you know if you are successful in meeting your career goals?

What is your timeframe?

Coaching Questions © 2019 The Nurse Leader Coach ™

PERSONAL MASTERY ASSESSMENT TOOLS FOR LEADER COACHES

Discover your own strengths by taking the ***Clifton Strength-finders*** assessment. Upon completion, you will receive a full report on your top five strengths and an insight guide on how to use your strengths. You can access this assessment by purchasing the Strengths-Based Leadership book in the chapter references which includes a code to take the assessment. You can also go online to the Gallup StrengthsFinder™ site to purchase a code https://www.gallupstrengthscenter.com/Purchase You may want to share the report with a trusted colleague.

Evaluate your emotional intelligence by doing the ***TalentSmart Emotional Intelligence Appraisal***. You can access this assessment by purchasing the book *Emotional Intelligence 2.0,* written by Travis Bradberry and Jean Greaves which includes a code to take the assessment. Upon completion, you will receive a customized report revealing your current skill levels and guidance about what you can do to improve. Commit yourself to improve in at least one of the four areas of emotional intelligence.

Personality plays a huge role in how we make decisions, handle responsibilities and form goals. As a coach, you need to decode your personality before you work with others because it has a strong influence on your coaching. The five-factor OCEAN model is an easy to use roadmap that can be used to assess your personality and that of others. Assess yourself on the five factors that are part of the OCEAN model (openness, conscientiousness extraversion, agreeableness, and neuroticism. The ***five-factor personality test*** is available for free at https://www.123test. com/big-five-personality-theory/

READ AND LISTEN TO LEAD – FREE RESOURCES

Hospitals and Health Networks Hospitals and Health Networks is published by Health Forum and is the official publication of the American Hospital Association. Free digital and magazine subscriptions are available for nurse leaders. The publication covers a wide range of healthcare leadership topics. Podcast interviews with health leaders are also available on the site. http://www.hhnmag.com/

SmartBrief on Leadership SmartBrief on Leadership provides various articles and blog postings related to innovative ideas about leadership and management. Users can subscribe and updates will be sent directly through e-mail. https://www2.smartbrief.com/signupSystem/subscribe.action?pageSequence=1&briefName=leadership&utm_source=brief

Fierce Healthcare Fierce Healthcare is a daily newsletter that is a leading source of healthcare management news. This is an excellent resource for nurse leaders on a wide range of healthcare leadership topics. Subscriptions are free. http://www.fiercehealthcare.com/

Kaiser Health News Kaiser Health News (KHN) is a nonprofit news organization committed to in-depth coverage of health care policy and politics of interest to healthcare leaders. A free email news subscription is available. http://kaiserhealthnews.org/

Emerging RN Leader Website Author: Dr. Rose O Sherman, EdD, RN, FAAN posts twice weekly posts (Monday and Thursday) on leadership topics targeted to developing healthcare and nursing leaders. Many blogs include free leadership resources. www.emergingrnleader.com

Institute for Health Care Improvement Open School The IHI is internationally recognized for work in quality improvement. They now have an open school on the internet that is used by many universities and health systems. This site contains 19 foundational courses on patient-and family-centered care, quality improvement, patient safety, managing healthcare operations, and leadership for a modest subscription fee. http://www.ihi.org/education/ihiopenschool/Pages/default.aspx

Harvard Business Review Ideacast The HBR IdeaCast, from the publishers of Harvard Business Review, Harvard Business Press, and hbr.org, features breakthrough ideas and commentary from the leading thinkers in business and management. These are weekly podcasts and you can subscribe to them for free on Itunes. https://itunes.apple.com/podcast/hbr-ideacast/id152022135?mt=2

Read to Lead Podcast This is a weekly leadership podcast built on the philosophy that the best leaders are readers. Jeff Brown interviews authors of the newest leadership books and discusses key learnings from the books. https://readtoleadpodcast.com/

Coaching for Leaders Podcast This is an excellent weekly podcast hosted by Dave Stachowiak who interviews some of the best leadership thinkers and coaches. Dave founded his podcast with the belief that leaders are not born—they are made and leadership skills can be learned. https://coachingforleaders.com/

TED TALKS FOR
NURSE LEADER COACHES

What if a short 15-20-minute video could capture the essence of a very creative person's thinking on a challenging topic? Well, there are such videos out there. The good news is that they are free–known as TED Talks. TED is a nonprofit devoted to ideas worth spreading. It started in 1982 as a conference bringing together people from three worlds: **Technology, Entertainment, Design.** TED Talks are on a wide range of topics with some related to personal experiences, and others such as The TED Talks on leadership focused specifically on leadership topics. These talks can be accessed at https://www.ted.com/talks. The following are some of my favorite TED Talks that I believe every nurse leader coach should watch:

The Puzzle of Motivation – Daniel Pink
Career analyst Dan Pink examines the puzzle of motivation, starting with the fact that social scientists know but most managers don't. Traditional rewards aren't always as effective as we think. Every coach should watch this.

How Great Leaders Inspire Action – Simon Sinek
Simon Sinek has a simple but powerful model for nurse leader coaches all starting with a golden circle and the question "Why?"

The Power of Introverts – Susan Cain
In a culture where being social and outgoing are prized above all else, it can be difficult, even shameful, to be an introvert. But, as Susan Cain argues in this passionate talk, introverts bring extraordinary talents and abilities to the world and should be encouraged and celebrated. If you are an introverted nurse leader coach, you will want to watch this video.

Dare to Disagree – Margaret Heffernan

Most people instinctively avoid conflict, but as Margaret Heffernan shows us, reasonable disagreement is central to progress. She illustrates (sometimes counterintuitively) how the best partners aren't echo chambers, and how great research teams, relationships, and businesses allow people to disagree constructively. Managing conflict well is essential to being a great coach.

The Surprising Habits of Original Thinkers – Adam Grant

Organizational psychologist, Adam Grant, studies creative people who come up with new ideas. What he found out about creative people may shatter some of your beliefs and make you a better coach.

What Makes Us Feel Good About our Work – Dan Ariely

What motivates us to work? Contrary to conventional wisdom, it isn't just money. However, it's not exactly joy either. It seems that most of us thrive by making constant progress and feeling a sense of purpose. Behavioral economist Dan Ariely presents two eye-opening experiments that reveal our unexpected and nuanced attitudes toward meaning in our work. A must for nurse leader coaches.

SAMPLE NEW NURSE LEADER COACH DEVELOPMENT PLAN

CHOOSE ONE GOAL IN EACH DOMAIN

Coaching Domain	Goal	Action Steps	Desired Outcomes	Timeframe
Building a Coaching Foundation	Gain Trust with My Staff	• Schedule meetings with all my direct reports to determine what is going well on the unit, what needs to change, what are their unique strengths and what do they expect of you. • Request a leader-mentor in my organization to provide guidance. • Avoid making any major changes initially in my new role.	• Begin deposits into the emotional trust piggybank. • Begin to build psychological safety on the unit. • Learn about the uniqueness of each staff member – their strengths, goals, and expectations.	June – September

Developing Your Coach Skills	Improve our Gallup Q12 Engagement Scores	• Identify the two lowest scoring items in Q12 questions 1-6. • Share the Q12 results at a staff meeting and seek feedback. • Develop three improvement strategies to implement in the 2 lowest scoring areas.	• Increase engagement scores on the questions by 20%. • Involve staff in developing initiatives to improve engagement.	Use October Q12 Results October–March
Coaching Teams to Higher Performance	Develop a unit-based staff recognition program.	• Select at least three award nominations that you will submit staff members for each year. • Survey all your direct reports to ask how they would like to be recognized. • Write two thank you notes to staff each week to thank them for above and beyond performance.	• Recognize professional and team excellence. • Provide individualize recognition that is meaningful to each staff member. • Encourage the heart through recognition of small contributions to patient care and teamwork.	December–January, and Ongoing

© 2019 The Nurse Leader Coach ™

ABOUT THE AUTHOR

Rose O. Sherman, EdD, RN, NEA-BC, FAAN is nationally known for her work in helping current and future nurse leaders to develop their leadership and coaching skills. Rose is a professor of nursing administration and financial leadership at Florida Atlantic University in Boca Raton Florida. She received a BA in Political Science and BSN in Nursing from the University of Florida. Her Master's Degree in Nursing is from the Catholic University of America, and she has a doctorate in nursing leadership from Columbia University in New York City. Before becoming a faculty member, she had a twenty-five-year nursing leadership career with the Department of Veterans Affairs at five VA Medical Centers.

Rose edits a popular leadership blog, www.emergingrnleader.com which is read by thousands of nurses each week. She also serves as editor in chief of *Nurse Leader*, the official journal of the American Organization of Nurse Executives. Her research work has been published in more than 90 peer-reviewed journals. She is a fellow in the American Academy of Nursing and alumni of the Robert Wood Johnson Executive Nurse Fellowship Program. Rose is a Gallup Certified Strengths Coach. In 2018, she received the Nurse Researcher of the Year award from the

AONE foundation. Rose has done individual leader coaching and presented on leadership and coaching topics for numerous health systems and professional organizations. She can be reached at roseosherman@outlook.com.

BRING THE NURSE LEADER COACH™ PROGRAM TO YOUR ORGANIZATION

Retaining nurses is challenging in today's competitive job market. Nurse turnover rates are increasing, replacement costs are extremely high, and the quality of care is threatened. Nurse leaders play a crucial role in staff retention. The contemporary nursing workforce has different expectations of their managers. What nurses want are leader coaches who focus on their performance development. Effective coaching is strengths-based, engagement focused and performance oriented. A failure to provide this results in lower staff engagement and higher turnover. Moving from being a traditional nurse leader to becoming a leader coach requires a new skill set and leadership approach. Just telling nurse leaders to do more coaching is not enough. The Nurse Leader Coach™ skill pre-assessment and workshop is an innovative, affordable program designed to equip your leaders with practical coaching methods and tools that can immediately be applied in the work setting. The goal is to help managers make coaching a regular part of their leadership practice. In addition to the coaching workshop, individual nurse leader coaching packages are also available. You can learn more by contacting Rose O. Sherman at roseosherman@outlook.com

Made in the USA
Middletown, DE
20 November 2024

65082193R00137